YOUR NATURAL BEAUTY HAIR AND SKIN CARE GUIDE

Best All-Natural Products, Simple Homemade Recipes, Natural Beauty Tips & Tricks and more

Table of Contents

INTRODUCTION

Hair care and skin care is and will always be a hot topic, and it is not shocking how are more and more people going to lines and therapies for natural skin and hair care with such excitement and debate over the ever more popular synthetic ingredients used in today's products. Natural hair and skin remedies continue to become more popular on the market, and with more and more consumers opting for these more natural treatments, you will soon be able to find different kinds of cosmetics for all your beauty care needs.

People are healthy enough, yet at a young age, they have split hair and hair loss. A positive sign of good health is nourished hair. Give your hair the right treatment. Leave your hair (and skin!) as tidy as you can. ***Rule no.1 Do not use heavy chemicals in your beauty care!*** A balanced lifestyle is a secret to a perfectly stunning and healthy appearance.

Hair and skin care should be taken; **naturally**! Coloring, grooming, and poor diet are all causes that can be linked to hair injury and bad skin conditions. A variety of things you should take into account to enhance your hair's overall look and health of your skin by providing the body with vital vitamins and minerals that contribute to a healthier lifestyle and these natural beauty care tips can quickly leave poor hair days behind. *"Hair stirs sight, touch, and scent sensations and memories — it's arousing and primal in its appeal."* Women spend hours at the hairdresser and beauty shops just to be seen as a beauty goddess. Nonetheless, you can have a beautiful hair without having to go to luxurious rooms, and the hairdryer saves hours. In this book you will discover how to fix your most annoying hair problems as well how to nourish and detox your skin!

CHAPTER ONE

The Psychology of Beauty

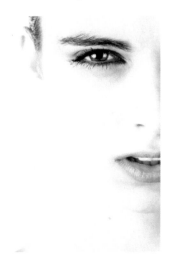

<u>The various attractiveness myths and the role of interpretation in determining appearance.</u>

The perception of attractiveness is complicated not just because the concept of attractiveness is unclear but also because beauty is most real in the mind of the viewer or in the way people view others. Beauty can be related to anything that is consistent with our senses and with all things. Beauty, as we see it, is essentially a reflection of our needs and beautiful objects or individuals, which simply satisfies our ideas or imaginations and represents our innate desire to connect to all that is appealing. People are guided by the senses, and we prefer to imitate processes and interactions which are harmonious, structurally, and formally pleasing to the senses. Appearance demands our sense of sight such that the feeling of appearance is expected to be replicated.

Yet **how do we see the beauty, and why are certain individuals or artifacts more attractive than others?** In the interpretation of appearance, psychological assessments found symmetry and proportion to be highly significant. Beauty is also more abstract than descriptive as a lovely product is evaluated as a complete item that is not measured according to its components but appealing. Freudian and psychoanalytic theories of beauty are rare, but psychoanalytic definitions may be viewed as interpretations or fulfillments of our perception of beauty, including individuals who would typically respect or serve our own desires. Psychoanalysis may also be consistent with the concept of desire for appearance if parent-like expectations are detected. Many men are often found pretty because they have a baby face or other innocence. Beauty may also be culturally influenced, so women with pretty feet are found sexy in many eastern societies, while in England, in the Victorian era, women with beauty and grace were measured by their limits, their lower body, and their eyes. The definition of appearance can vary, and studies have shown that women can choose softer characteristics for men at certain periods and more masculine characteristics at certain times due to the point of their breeding cycles.

Eventually, beauty is how we see the natural world and how we turn our desires and expectations into what we see beyond. Appearance in the eyes of the beholder' is absolutely mentally right because the time and our desires, esthetic sense, and interpretation of appearance alter our own tastes.

Natural Beauty

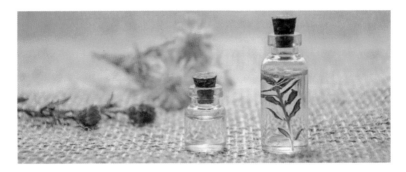

Would you love to go to Bora Bora, but don't have time? Maybe you and your love will find relaxation, harmony, and intimate moments by creating a 'spa' at home. It is one of my favorite things to do! It's not for you until you know. Spa times are about mingling together. This is a low risk - high effect that spices up your life and shifts tension dynamics. Gather the supplies over the week, schedule a time for children to play, and take out the coupons you have made for Anniversary Day.

You would enjoy those minutes of rest as you take the time to spend a day full of the mind and body as a human being. There's a beautiful thing about a fragrant bath full of salts and dried herbs, lotions that reach deep into the skin and allow the general glow of feeling good and hydrated. There is nothing more beautiful in the world than in this glistening place of relaxation confidence. The slow pace of life will turn into a slow wake with the one you love if you wish.

I want to share my "secrets of beauty" so I can pamper myself too. It's a global human phenomenon. People also love the spa day. Most families nowadays tend to cool down, to see friends. But my honey and me... we try to spend a decent time dreaming, chatting, and calming.

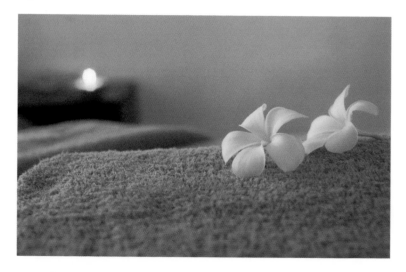

Therapeutic contact It may seem an odd way to start the day. I use aromatherapy oil and the house's quietness to enable him to relieve the tension between his feet, bald heads, and especially his arms and necks, behind his ears. This isn't as much a massage as a soft caress. It's a nice moment of mutual reconciliation for all of us. Use it as a prelude to your spa day with your loved one and set the stage for relaxing.

Natural, nature...There's always intrinsic happiness now that there is inner peace: natural beauty. You may need to be mindful of this since some specialty shopping is necessary. Be imaginative. Be innovative. Any of these items are available in a natural food store. And lots of natural beauty tips for spa day can be found online.

As in a salon, you want to mold your hair profoundly and then gently. It is a wonderful service received by the National Honey Board. (https://www.honey.com)

The extremes of heat and cold we experience all winter will make even the biggest of hair look and smell like straw. This **herbal conditioner** mixes honey with shine, moisture olive oil, and Rosemary essential oil to promote hair growth.

1/2 cup Honey 1/4 cup of warmed Rosemary 1 tsp. Essential oils four drops of olive oil (2T for fine to oily hair). Place all the ingredients in a bowl and blend thoroughly in the xanthan gum (available in health food stores). Place the close-fitting stopper or deck in a clean plastic container. Apply a minimal volume to mildly humidified hair at a time. Massage scalp and hair combination until completely powdered. Cover hair with a moist towel (microwave towel or dryer may be heated) or a shower cap; let nourish and set aside for 30 minutes. Remove towel or shower cap; gently wash and clean with cold water. Dry as usual and enjoy the natural way of shinier, smoother, and healthier hair.

If you've comfortably blended that with your tresses, you obviously complement the mask with Rose Oil and Honey. The recipe comes from the National Honey Board as well (https://www.honey.com). This mask will clean your skin and replenish it. Sweet and quickly consumed, light almond oil softens and feeds the flesh. Honey will moisturize your skin.

Ready to clean and exfoliate the skin? This Share Ambrosia remedy is excellent as a body wash.

It is a peppermint-twisting Honey Almond wash! This treatment exfoliates the skin to make it cleaner and smoother.

Ingredients: 4 t almond oil, 2 t Jojoba oil, 4 T Honey, 5 drops of Peppermint essential oil in a 4 oz cobalt or amber glass container (preferably) add into the almond and Jojoba oil. Heat well.. Then add in the essential oil of Honey and Peppermint. Continue to stir until the mixture is thoroughly blended.

To use: first, cleanse the flesh. Apply the scrub on a wet face around a tablespoon. To make it more flexible (don't apply water to the jar), combine with water. Scrub the skin gently and let the almond meal do the job (harder pressure will hurt the capillaries!). Massage per centimeter of skin with the exception of the fragile tissue of the eye. Remove a wet washcloth. Cover. Be aware that any piece of the scrub is eliminated. To extract excess liquid, apply a tonic or hydrosol with a cotton pad. Finish with the use of the humidifier. Using about once a week to keep the skin moist and smooth and to alleviate surface pain.

Soaking bath salts is my sanctuary. The best salt you can blend conveniently at home.

My recipe: Combine a bottle of Epsom salts with a .5-ounce healthy oil from your preferred skin that is usually purchased in a candle store, baths, or craft market. I order my essential oils and aromatherapy online, and it's easy to find them. I use a deep ceramic roasting pan to combine all of our salts in a small batch and then allow them to dry several hours until they can be put on the market for quarter glass bottles.

My favorite addition is dried flowers, which I cut into and remove from mildew in a warm oven. A special oil blend contributes to the soaking process of whole herbs, roses, and carnations. Remove the stem, but the flowers on the basis; if you cut roses, ensure that the rosehip is in your drying bowl. Thanks to the soothing value of milk to the flesh, you should even apply dried milk to your blend.

Don't hesitate to use candles openly and turn off hard lights in your home. Select your favorite calming scents.

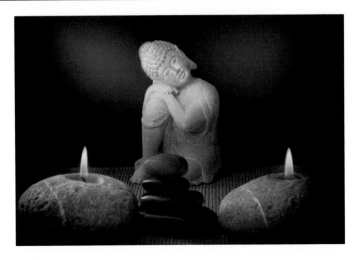

I'm very generous about the use of bath salts, so I'm going to sprinkle a full-size bath with two or three cups, including vitamin E, so occasionally lavender oil, if my soul is involved. I using the fragrance of the Dragon's Bloodflower most frequently in the shower, but I recently added even an essential oil blend of patchouli and lavender and aromatherapy for the headaches, etc. The Epsom salts are perfect for restful pains and soreness in the body.

It is important to remember that none of this concentrate is "edible," even if it consists of typical ingredients. They can stay in the refrigerator more comfortably and can be in a securely packed container.

Adapt your life to it.

When your partner is hesitant, and you have children at home, make it a day of play for them. I had some fun time recently.. Six women had been out overnight, and the most fun thing in towels was toenail polish, honey face, and hair. It was amazing!!

Adapt it all to your personality.

Bring that happy moment in your life. Make it happen for yourself. ***You must be your own support and you must respect yourself for your own mental health***.

Enjoy a nice cup of tea, humor, and meaningful talk while you relax. Stop the electronics for the day; disconnect the machine and the phone. In this world of rushing, it is vital that you take time to invest, particularly in your wife or husband, friend, or family member. Relax, and just focus on these emotions of thanks and affection. A short ride to the nearest bath and body will offer many of the same items, as well as the healthier variations of the organic food market.

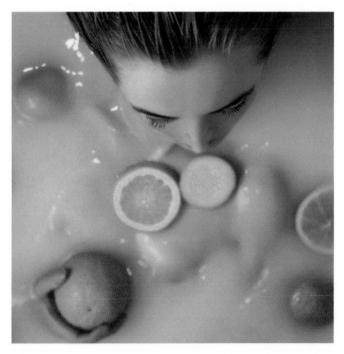

Natural Beauty Hair Care Information

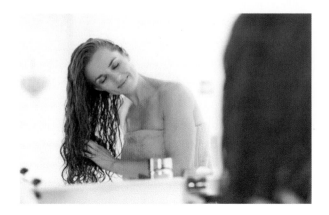

As I have mentioned earlier, haircare is and will still be a hot subject, and it is not shocking that more and more consumers are turning toward natural beauty hair care products and treatments despite some excitement and debate over the ever more popular synthetic ingredients used in today's products.

Natural hair remedies continue to become more popular on the market, and with more and more consumers opting for these more natural treatments, you will soon be able to find different kinds of cosmetics for all your hair care needs.

Natural skin and hair care for most people is not necessarily a top priority. Many people have made so many choices about shampoo aisles, conditioners, gels, mousses, and other hair care products that it is impossible to determine what to choose and what should really be off from their list.

Too many customers are puzzled and upset about which safe and organic goods to choose for new products on the market. Here you can find a few tips to help you choose a natural beauty hair care product, and these tips can hopefully help you get rid of some of the confusion of finding hair care products in general.

Tip #1. Learn the packaging - goods containing tons of organic additives can be easily found from looking at the backs of the products. The longer the names and the less pronounceable the names, the more industrial ingredient is. There are a number of botanical names and medicinal names in the ingredient list of natural products. So these botanical names would be as prominent as possible on the register. Unless these are the last mentioned ingredients, so perhaps not much of the ingredient is used in the finished product.

Tip #2. Avoid everything under the form of "paraben." Paraben is preservatives, and while preservatives are required in your items of natural beauty, paraben is not the best route to be maintained. Paraben has a full list of adverse side effects, so it is safe to remove them from beauty products.

Tip #3. When you have questions, find out product reports online. Too many recommendations can be found online that there is no need to pick items randomly because they look or smell fine. Have a look and see the top natural product creators, including Origins (https://www.origins.com) or Burt's Bees (https://www.burtsbees.co.uk/) By merely browsing Google, you will find hundreds of items for any need you face.

Tip #4. Consider alternative natural elegance to the use of processed goods. Products such as carrier oils and essential oils are also readily accessible online, and others can be conveniently added without the difficulty of working with a range of products in your makeup routine. The site features some excellent posts on natural beauty to assist with a variety of health issues.

As you can see, you can quickly reduce the chances of adding dangerous or potentially hazardous goods in life by following any of these guidelines.

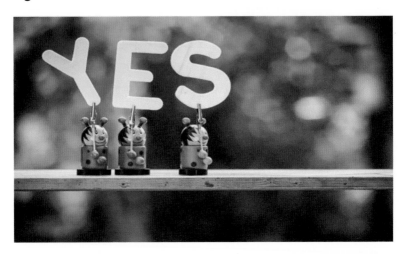

Best All-Natural Products

We live in a world with preservatives and goods that we can't even start pronouncing with a long list of ingredients. Thankfully, we don't have to live like that. We have other options for the goods we purchase. You don't have to be packed with chemicals and other stuff that only hurt our bodies. We can all begin to live a healthy, organic, chemical life.

One of the first ways to begin your new organic life is through the purchase of organic items such as organic lotions. These products will only contain natural ingredients and will be organically grown and will be safer for the body. For example, for lotions, preservatives and harmful chemicals often found in other lotions are not present in the best organic lotions. Therefore, organic products are particularly beneficial for those with sensitive skin. Some of the chemical compounds used in non-organic lotions and other cosmetics are causing skin irritation and can cause more serious problems. Although these other products have caused the issues, the best organic lotions will help reduce the effects of skin conditions and issues.

However, you don't have to quit using organic cosmetics. In all facets of your life, you should go organically. A second place to go is to only purchase organic goods. Organic products were produced without traditional pesticides or chemical fertilizers. The food was not packed with chemical ingredients. Natural products are often harvested separately from other products not organically grown. It eliminates the possibility of combining the organic with non-organically grown products.

There is also no limit on how much your life can be free of organic and chemical substances. If you haven't already begun, begin with something little and get away from it. You will lead a healthy organic and chemical-free life.

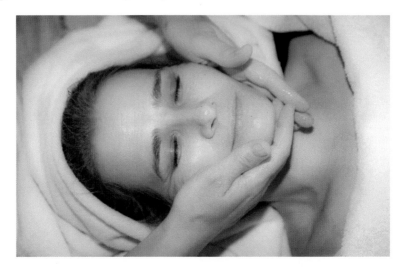

Hair We Grow Again

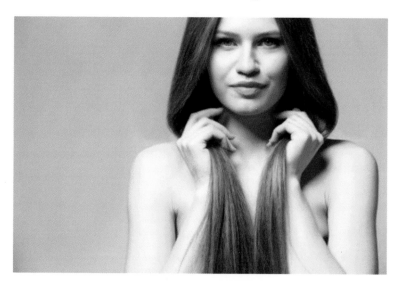

Today we have not only to overcome the usual problems of good hair, and there are toxins in the air; bleach additives and preservatives that contribute to the misery of our food.

Let us first look at the causes of bad hair:

- Zinc Deficiency
- Poor nutrition
- Yeast Infections
- Fungus
- Stress
- High use of alkaline shampoo
- Thyroid Disease
- Iron Deficiency

NUTRITION Though consuming plenty of water and eating foods rich in vitamins and minerals is vital for wellbeing, and there are other supplements necessary for good and lovely hair. Omega3, vitamins

A, B, C, D, F, magnesium, calcium, selenium, phosphorus, and alpha-linoleic acid are all fatty acids.

OMEGA-3 FATTY ACIDS Fatty acids Omega-3 are important for the hair follicles, as they are tougher, shinier, and quicker. Omega-3 fatty acid deficiency can lead to a dry scalp.

VITAMIN A Vitamin A is an essential part of hair growth and survival and encourages a healthy scalp. For smooth, well-conditioned hair, a good scalp is important. The production of retinoic acid in the hair follicle is regulated as well. This facilitates the development of sebum along with vitamin C, which is secreted by hair follicles and acts as a natural hair conditioner. This may be taken indoors or immediately applied to the hair shaft and massaged into the scalp.

Vitamin A is a big component of the sweet potatoes, lettuce, cabbage, cantaloupe, butter, dried apricots, mozzarella cheese, mango.

VITAMIN B Tension is known to induce loss of hair. Vitamin B not only helps to relieve tension in the body but one of the B vitamins, Inositol, has proven that hair growth is quick. B12 also helps reduce hair loss because it is a hair factor. B vitamins are best obtained as B-complexes combined.

Foods like rice, whole grain, onions, lettuce, oranges contain B vitamins.

VITAMIN C Iron is also essential for hair growth, and vitamin C allows the body to absorb iron. For the development of collagen, vitamin C is essential for the preservation and repair of connective tissue. Hair follicles contain collagen-rich connective tissue. Because the body does not produce its own vitamin C, diets and supplements are the only way to get it.

Lemons, limes, rose hips, beans, tomatoes, chocolate, onions, Brussels sprouts and broccoli, all of which are high in vitamin C. The daily intake of vitamin C is recommended for 1000 to 2000 mg daily.

VITAMIN D Vitamin D activates the hair follicle and cells that minimize hair loss for the hair shaft. Vitamin D deficiency can lead to flaccid scalp and psoriasis. And, as we know, for healthy hair, a healthy scalp is important. Vitamin D is also especially important as it stimulates the hair shaft and scalp.

Vitamin D rich foods include soy yogurt, yogurt, orange juice, and cereals.

VITAMIN E Nutrient E is a major nutrient for wellbeing and beauty in your face. It ensures that your scalp's blood circulates normally, and it is a fat-soluble vitamin that improves your hair's shine as it grows. Deficiencies can make the hair brittle and dull.

Increased consumption can be accomplished with a vitamin E supplement or with the addition of raw nuts and peas, beans, wheat germ oil, and green leafy vegetables to your everyday diet.

ZINC has important antioxidant properties for the immune system. This helps avoid other kinds of hair loss by stimulating hair follicles.

Zinc-containing foods such as pumpkin seeds, dark chocolate, garlic, seeds of sesame, wheat germ, and chickpeas.

IRON Low iron levels can cause anemia. Since anemia may have underlying causes, such as hyperthyroidism, which are known to cause hair loss, iron is essential to combat the anemic thyroid influence.

High-in-iron diet contains black, leafy vegetables, nuts, grains and iron-enriched rice, beans, lentils, chickpeas, soybeans, and artichoke.

SELENIUM Selenium is an antioxidant that allows the body to rid itself of the adverse effects of the sun and atmosphere radiation. It is also essential to support the capacity of your body to sustain proper functions such as hair growth and strengthen your immune system.

Selenium occurs in foods such as Brazilian nuts, sunflower seeds, whole grain, and onions, chocolate, garlic.

ALPHA-LINOLEIC ACID Alpha-linoleic acid, like Omega-3, is an essential fatty acid. It creates a shield against moisture depletion on our hair and serves as a conditioner. Fatty acids have also been shown to enhance hair growth.

Alpha-linoleic acid sources contain flaxseeds, flaxseed oil, canola oil, soya oil, pumpkin seeds, pumpkin seed oil, perilla oils, tofu, walnuts, and walnut butter.

To add to the requirement to consume a healthy diet that contains these and other nutritional supplements, the rest will, of course, be consumed orally in the form of vitamins. Natural ingredients may also be used on the hair in order to preserve their beauty and health.

Like natural vitamins and indoor supplements for healthy, picturesque beauty, the best must be used externally too.

HAIR PRODUCTS Many shampoos contain additives that are harmful to the hair. Examples include sodium lauryl sulfate, ammonium lauryl sulfate, ammonium lauryl sulfate, ammonium xylene sulfonate, TEA lauryl sulfate, sulfur in shampoo dandruff, and selenium sulfides. You may opt to read all of the labels in-store, take a list (with more ingredients than this), or find homeopathic/natural shampoos to save time to aggravation. Sunlight, toxins, blow-drying, and coloring continue to strip the hair of the natural oils.

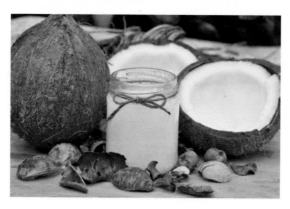

COCONUT OIL Coconut oil is a safe and easy treatment for the wellbeing of scalp and hair. The high saturated fat content of the coconut oil includes medium-chain triglycerides that are well associated with the hair structure, according to Organic Evidence. Virgin cocoa oil is the strongest, as it retains its antioxidant properties, and even vitamins E and K. Coconut oil provide vitality and liveliness to your hair while keeping your scalp clean and lice and egg-free hair.

BIOTIN, also known as Vitamin H, a member of the B-complex community, contributes to the energy transition of food into a healthy hair. Biotin avoids hair loss and dried and scaly skin, which is attributed to Biotin defects caused by seborrheic dermatitis. Biotin preserves hair resilience and durability by battling fracturing and torn hair.

TEA TREE OIL Tea Tree Oil, a native of Australia, has a wide variety of uses, including clothing, for general wellbeing and wellness. The antiseptic effects help to eliminate the hair shaft buildup caused by water salts and the application of chemical products. It also eliminates pelvic and unhealthy dead cells on the skin and helps clear damaged hair follicles that normalize the pH equilibrium in the hair so that impaired hair will re-grow.

LAVENDAR OIL Lavender Oil is also known as Tea Tree Oil for its anti-fungal and antiseptic properties. This destroys not only bacteria and fungi, which can cause dandruff and hair loss but also has significant effects and improves hair shine.

Homeopathic Arnica can be used as an up-to-date cream or in shampoos and conditioners, when used in stressful conditions, that cause abundant itching and skin flaking. Topical creams work rapidly as they are immediately applied to the scalp. Pregnant women cannot use Arnica because it can stimulate the uterus.) After all, lovely hair must be protected from the inside. (Warning-Arnica, suspected to be toxic when swallowed, can result in heart arrest and death. All the organic products, shampoos, oils, and coatings do not do a thing well if there is not enough in the body to build and support good and lovely hair. However, so-called beauty products that do more harm than good, so natural products are better used to care for your hair.

CHAPTER TWO

What Can You Do About Hair Loss?

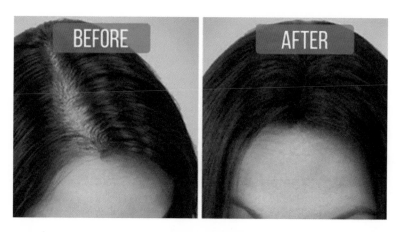

A good friend was recently really concerned about her hair loss. It happens that she gave a birth to a gorgeous baby, and hair loss after birth occurs in few cycles.

Indeed, it is part of a pattern, since women's hair becomes thicker and thinner during pregnancy, but it is also shorter and keep loses just the same after birth. This condition can be extended to six months. Then the hair will gradually and naturally return to its usual period of development.

We lose around 100 hairs a day on average! Normally, we find this when we wash or comb the hair. The hair grows for 2-6 years, about half an inch every month. Then take a two to three-month rest time and finally continue to slide. According to scientists, 10% of the hair is now still, and the remaining 90% is that.

Alopecia areata is a skin condition arising where the hair is small, and holes or "patches" are created. It is autoimmune, indicating that the body loses healthy body tissue in mistake. In most cases, the hair develops absolutely missing in some.

This condition typically develops in individuals with prior family background. It impacts 1.7% of the world's population (5 million U.S. residents).

Many disorders that may induce hair loss include thyroid issues, diabetes, lupus, side effects of prescription (such as some acne and lithium medications used for treatments for depressive disturbance), side effects of cancer treatments, such as chemical therapy, pain, bad diet (which does not consume enough protein, for example). People with anorexia and bulimia are typically affected by hair loss if they do not feed well.

Besides these diseases, the overuse of the hairdryer may also cause hair damage.

Hair loss solutions: If you're worried about hair loss, contact the doctor to investigate the potential causes first. The doctor will recommend a multivitamin from a chronic disorder or from an inadequate diet to help the case.

In comparison, if your hair drops fear, you should take the following tips, but not exaggerated:

1. Clean your hair softly.
2. Distort the hair with a small tooth comb and a cream, especially if your hair is thin and easily tangled.

3. Whenever practicable, dry your natural hair, and if you have nothing but a hand hairdryer, like to have a cooler temperature than usual.
4. Consider having ponytails or close braids before you resume your hair.
5. Using shampoo boy.
6. Stop brushing your hair too hard against the towel.

5 Tips to Have Naturally Beautiful Hair

The hair of a woman is also one of the first things that anyone can see as they look at her. It was said that the beauty of a woman is her crowning glory. It only makes sense to watch over your hair to see it in its beauty throughout the world. You should do a lot to maintain the natural elegance of your hair, aside from lavish therapies and trips to the salon.

#1. Remember first what you take into your body. Your hair represents pretty much what you're in. A healthy, nutritious diet guarantees a radiant head of hair like every shampoo or conditioner should provide. Your hair care is 1/4 hydration, and it's always nice to have 8-10 glasses of water a day. A healthy intake will enhance your hair, but it can also be affected by poor intake. Keep away from chemicals, cigarettes, and other toxic substances because they can adversely harm health.

_#2._ Use a towel for 10 minutes after the hair is dry to remove much of the moisture. Then remove the towel and allow your hair to dry at room temperature. Use a low heat blow dryer is good, but most moisture will be automatically dried out. This also helps combat hair hurt.

#3. You will also have a leg to prevent damage if you choose the right hairbrush. Seek to use larger pebbles to avoid touching the base wherever possible. Do not use a brush or comb to damage the hair while it is still wet. This breaks down your hair.

#4. Removing dry and fuzzy ends can continue to minimize damage, even as removing a faulty thread on your clothes removes further damage. Turn the hair downwards gently until the split ends appear. Using sharp haircutting shears to separate the broken ends carefully. Seek to keep it just to prevent a task.

#5. Proper shampoos and treatments and soft cosmetics are the perfect way to keep your hair healthy and happy. Choosing a fine, all-natural shampoo to cleanse deeply keep your hair follicles intruded in dirt and oils and preserve your skin smooth. The state is deep, as it preserves some of the washing moisture lost. Your hair contains oils on your scalp naturally and cleans these oils correctly without any dirt.

Taking into consideration, these five simple tips will go a long way to keep your hair clean and shiny. With a healthy lifestyle, cooking right, and treating your beauty as it belongs, the shine will be beautiful for everyone to see.

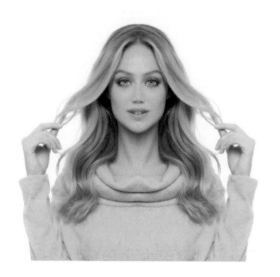

How to Co-Wash Natural Hair

Whether you're wearing natural color or not, you either know how to co-wash your hair using just conditioner. Conditioner brushing avoids unpleasant effects from repeated bathing of shampoos and helps keep natural black hair smooth and controllable. Co-washing should be done as much as you want, sometimes many times a day (this is a bonus in the humid summer days for natural hair users).

The question **"Why do I co-wash my hair?"** also emerges. The solution is easy, but several steps should be taken to make the best of this method and do it quickly.

__ Find your hairstyle conditioner.__* Check for "hair type" keywords online and narrow your hair type down to a similar category or two. You can be 3c and 4a mix. It will allow you to consider the sort of conditioner you should purchase from the others.

__ Choose your products.__* The long, difficult to foresee components on the label can be daunting. Yet you will know from experience what ingredients you want to keep and what you want to remove. Propylene glycol, acetyl alcohol, and pantheon are typical ingredients.

__*Recommended:*__ buy an extended head/tube toilet. Handheld shower heads with customizable sprays have the greatest leverage for hair rinsing and always worth investing.

__ Hair clean with warm water.__* Avoid water that's too hot. The action of water and purifier (shampoo and/or conditioner) and friction (hand gestures through the hair) results in purification.

Coldwater cleanses well the hair though ice water can be toxic. Wet your hair softly with your fingertips as you rinse with water.

Apply your conditioner. Here are some tips how to:

(1) Give your hand a line of conditioner (unlike pouring a dollop) and add each line on the section of your hair. Function from the roots to the tips of the conditioner. Try to cover all the hair.

(2) Squeeze the usual volume of conditioner, preferably acrylic, into a big tub. Apply water to the tub and mix the water and the conditioner well with your fingertips. Scoop up some of the mixes with a cup or other small jar and spill it onto your head. Then you can lean back into the tub and wash your hair directly over the pot. This makes further coverage feasible, but remember that the conditioner is diluted.

(3) Into a big, clean spray bottle, squeeze the usual amount of conditioner, and blend with water. Shake well and brush on your hair openly. Once, this combination will dilute rather than add directly. It is a perfect approach for those who have just minutes to spare in the morning. Make a big batch of distilled conditioner and spray the hair after bathing.

*Pair the hair with a rounded-edge comb. Each move is optional because there is still debate about whether peeling when wet creates more hair harm than peeling while dry. Combining wetness will stretch the hair beyond the longest point and cause breakage; it has been said. Nevertheless, many people who has natural hair say that combing their hair when it is completely washed is the best time for them because their hair is smooth and folding, which results in less rupture. In any case, softly strip the hair by taking a small part at a time. The key aim is to conveniently tangle and spread the packaging equally.

*** *Keep the conditioner on your hair at least a couple of minutes.* ** Suggestion: At this time, both the steam from the shower and the conditioner will work on your hair. Give yourself a nice salt or sugar scrub while you clean your hair.

* Well rinse your head with warm water again. Ease the fingers in each segment while the water flows through to avoid any residual conditioners.

*** *Optional:* ** In this step, add your hair products — when your hair drips wet. Even people enjoy this method and assume that at this point, the strongest absorption is received. At least, once your product(s) are hot, it can be spread more uniformly in your hair.

*** *You can dry your hair in many ways...here are some tips;* **

(1) Wet towel. Stop rubbing your skin and hair at all times with a towel! Only brush your hair dry or take pieces and squeeze excess water into the towel.

(2) Turn and go. Turn and go. Place your towel over your back (shoulder to shoulder lengthwise). Take the lower corners of your towel and raise it nearly above your ear. Think of Batman's cape as he runs away from a big house! Move your head from side to side with the towel raised (ear to shoulder) and turn left (as no), shake excess water onto the towel. That's what I call the 'no contact' strategy. Alternatively, drying hair with a towel will extract chemicals that you have added right now, even helping to differentiate your freshly formed spirals. You want to bring the coils together to stop the friction. This technique is ideal for the warmer months, where you can spend longer stretches of moist hair.

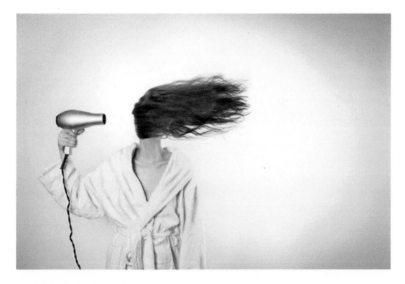

(3) _Dry off, but gently._ When blow-drying, it is safer to use a diffuser. A diffuser will uniformly spread the heat from your dryer and mitigate potential heat disruption. In most beauty supplies stores, diffusers are available at a low discount. If you do not have a diffuser, use the cold or low heat to blow dry from the farthest section of your hair at least six inches. Rest assured, you don't have to dry your hair — dry enough to style and leave.

In short, the above methods are an excellent alternative to conventional shampooing and will allow you to shampoo your hair with much-needed oils and moisture. Only a touch of preparation will take less than applying your makeup to and from the bathroom with a clean head of hair, and your beauty will benefit greatly.

The Benefits of Natural Skin, Hair, Bath and Body Products

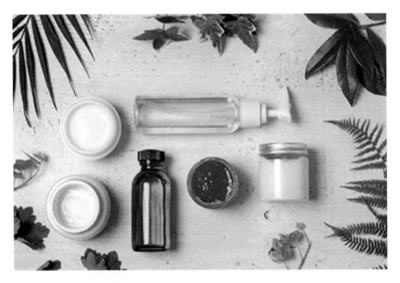

Most of us use toiletries and cosmetics in our lives for personal protection, grooming, or embellishment. Through our childhood years up to our dawning years, we continue with the use of rash creams, bubble bats, shampoos, oils, and talc's; perfumes, hair dyes, and cosmetics, after-shaves, creams, lotions, deodorants, bubble baths, shower gels, etc.

Unfortunately, all of these goods contain harmful substances, Skin, Hair, Bath, and Body, which can be poisonous and poisonous to our health. Many synthetic chemicals may be toxic, including allergic responses to the skin, imbalances in hormone, immune and nerve systems, infant development defects, and even cancer, are clear facts.

Since the skin is an absorbent organ, i.e., capable of absorbing what we place on it, it is important that we use items that are not toxic to our own health. Before you purchase the product, it will be prudent to raise your knowledge of unhealthy additives and read food labels.

The demand for natural goods is growing as more and more consumers become aware of the health concerns of common toiletries and cosmetics. Of which I mean finished products that are made from natural materials (which are often known to be natural chemicals), such as **shea butter, cocoon oil, sweet almond oil, plant extracts, essential oils**, etc. Neither man-made nor plastic are they. This phenomenon is also related to a broader problem of food poisoning, the air we breathe, drinking water, and the numerous ailments that may contribute to it.

Only to offer a fair perspective, even with natural materials, the question of health and toxicity is still there. Some people may induce allergic reactions, some are safe to use, but other people are just not safe to use in limited amounts. There is also a chance of degradation when poisons, insecticides, and air and water contaminants products enter the natural world.

Products like fats, butter, mineral oils, etc. can also be processed, distilled, or prepared in terms of the purity and strength of the ingredients. It is also essential for a distributor or retailer who uses quality materials to purchase your goods. The purest and most strong are raw, unrefined, or cold-pressed. Ask the manufacturer or retailer if you are confused and cannot find anything on the bottle. Any respectable and ethically based organization is prepared to share this material.

Given the health issues of natural goods, they are always my pick. Natural ingredients have much strong skin and body healing properties. Some ingredients are also holistic as they affect the human, body, mind, and feelings therapeutically. *Another source is Essential Oils, herbal products of various fauna and plants such as Lavender, Rose, and Chamomile.*

In my personal view, the production and use of natural Skin Care, Bath and Body products help me create a stronger bond with myself and Mother Earth, which can easily be missed living in a concrete, busy and lively city setting.

Cocoa Butter is perfect for the use of a very dry, dehydrated skin and chapped skin as it moisturizes, soothes, and preserves. Cocoa Butter is good skincare, a bathroom, and a body item. This is a good vitamin E source with many skin advantages. It is also prescribed for eczema, psoriasis, and dermatitis. It helps shield fragile skin from harmful conditions by building a moisture-resistant air barrier. Cocoa butter has a long tradition of being used by pregnant women to avoid and reduce stretch marks.

Evening Primrose Oil is an extremely nourishing treatment for dry, aged, or chapped skin when used externally. The high GLA helps to make the body tissue operate comfortably and may lead to disorders like eczema, psoriasis, fine lines, and wrinkles. This deals with diabetes, hypertension, breast tenderness, insomnia, eczema, elevated blood pressure, overweight, PMS internally.

Rose Essential Oil PMT and PMS, menopause symptoms, insomnia, hormonal sounds, pain, aphrodisiac, inflammation, tissue decongestion, bactericidal, control whole reproductive organs of females, refrigeration, impotence, uterine disorders, distress, post-natal depression, tonic to many species, for dry, responsive, mature skin. Great for delicate, dry, and healthy skin for small and young children.

Lavender Essential Oil regulates nerves, aches, and pain, rheumatic conditions, faintness, palpitation, stress and fatigue, depression, hydrogenation, highly antiseptic, toxic and cold conditions, high blood pressure, allergy, fog, bites, cuts, blisters, insomnia, eczema, acne, regulates scanty periods, cardiac regulator, asthma, bronchitis, epilepsy.

Honey is a natural humectant that allows moisture to be absorbed and maintained. The inherent moisturizing properties make it suitable for use in hydrating products. This is appropriate for allergic skin items as well. Studies have also shown that honey has significant natural antioxidant properties. Antioxidants help to shield the skin from UV exposure and to help rejuvenate the tissue. This is also antimicrobial and, therefore, beneficial for mild acne or contaminated skin areas (prevents the growth of such bacteria).

Aloe Vera is an important component that moisturizes, refrigerates, and soothes, particularly in After Sun products. It contains vitamin B complex, folic acid, vitamin C and carotene (the vitamin A precursor) oil, and has been derived from the Shea (Karite) nut, which has been used for natural skin and hair care in Africa for many centuries as cocoa butter. This is very moisturizing to help keep the skin intact and is beneficial for multiple skin conditions: dry, dehydrated and aging skin, improves the warm skin with eczema or psoriasis because it cures and soothes, is excellent for weakened skin (including stretch marks - a good component of pregnant belly balsam), preserves the skin of foreign elements.

The most common use of **_white kaolin (clay)_** is for delicate skin. Rich in coal. A soft, less absorbing clay which cleanses and clarifies the skin effectively. Softens and tones. Softens and tones.

Calendula can be particularly useful for delicate, dry, and advanced skin types as a herbal extract or as an oil infusion. Good for all skin conditions, eczema, psoriasis, chapping, dry or broken skin in particular. This is also beneficial to account for increased skin oil production and to heal cuts, scars, burns, inflammations, and other bruises as this help repair tissue. The oil that nourishes the skin and soothes inflamed skin, psoriasis, eczema, every form of dermatitis. May help regulate skin or scalp acne and oily, since excess sebum in jojoba dissolves.

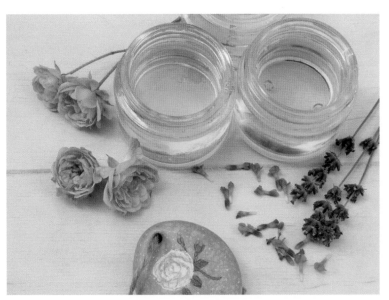

CHAPTER THREE

Natural Skin and Hair Care

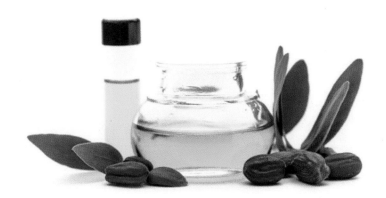

Why Natural?

What would you think if you see people running fuel through their hair and buying miniature bottles to use for hand and foot hydration while driving to your local gas station? Imagine if you see the workers leap into a massive jacuzzi on a visit to a chemical plant whose froth and bubbles were created by the remnants of what they had made the same day. No matter how little or how much you know of natural personal care goods, you would certainly not want to think that these goods advertise because of the way they were introduced to you.

Unfortunately, you slip into your shampoo, makeup, and lotion other ingredients. To add insults, these synthesizers are sold on the market in bottles that say "all-natural, botanical," and "clean." You will unwittingly feed your body's biggest, permeable organ, but daily doses of carcinogenic and harmful meals, unless you take the time to research and examine the ingredients used in your personal care items.

In addition to traditional purifiers and emulsions (e.g., lotions and creams), potentially dangerous chemicals include lauryl and laureth sulfates (surfactants and lathering agents that heat the skin and hair), and various parabens and PEG (petroleum compounds, potential carcinogenesis). The valuable by-product of the soap cycle is also extracted from bar soap and sold individually in order to help enhance the drying quality of the additives in the soap. Glycerin is a valuable by-product. Conditioners typically represent a toxic mixture that includes a small proportion of nutrient components, the effects of synthetic loss are needless, and the residual that causes the build-up of the substance needs every few months to turn to another substance. Household hot oil and other pre-wash therapies that can be left in other shampooed out to provide the most successful safe condition. There can be up to 200 different synthetic components in one fragrance spray! Basic oils are the only component to perfume a drug to use on human or animal bodies. Healthy preservatives include neem oil and extracts of rosemary and grapes.

The makeup industry is a multimillion-dollar business where the idea of using only pure and raw products to cultivate hair and skin builds traction slowly but steadily. However, other impostors and half-hearted attempts benefit from the alluring noise. That is why the following knowledge allows people to navigate the oceans, wherever the point they are in their quest for natural beauty.

SHAMPOOS, BAR, AND LIQUID SOAPS

Truly natural soap is made from fats and oils, with a solid base such as sodium or potassium hydroxide. The end result is soap and water, and the lye is usually used. The resulting substance is referred to as cold process soap, as this process happens at room temperature. Few natural soaps can be made with heat as well. Natural glycerin remains in the soap, and other herbal soapers incorporate botanical clays, herbs, and essential oils to improve the soap consistency. It results in a superior soap bar that purifies and nourishes the scalp. Natural liquid soaps may be used with skin and hair interchangeably. We advocate **Castile liquid soap** https://en.wikipedia.org/wiki/Castile_soap for both and sticking to preservative- and dyes-free labels. Many soapers have botanical mixtures that are especially good for the scalp.

CONDITIONERS AND BEAUTY PRODUCTS

Most conditioners operate well if their ingredients are clean. The therapies vary from hot oil treatment of mixed and essential oils, a mixture of clay and ground herbs to a fresh food mask that may contain ingredients including natural milk, ginger, avocado, and olive oil in your refrigerator. It it stays long enough (heat expands pores such that the product can be absorbed more quickly), even after the shampoo, the nutritional components of care remain. This helps you to achieve all the benefits of conditioning without thinking about drug development. *Aloe Vera Gel* is a perfect beauty mouse/gel that works from straight hair to dreadlocks. It works without making hair stiff and can also provide texture when it comes to hair styles, both straight and curly.

TONERS, EXFOLIATORS, AND MAKEUP PRODUCTS.

Floral waters and hydrosols are the mildest and most nourishing for the skin (by-products of the processing of essential oils). _Witch hazel_ is perfect for oily skin, for dry skin _lavender_, for aged skin _rose,_ and delicate _chamomile_. Effective exfoliators and moisturizing agents for the body are oil-based sugar and salt scrubbing. To exfoliate the skin, using apricot and fresh pureed papaya or pineapple (or masks containing such enzymes as an alternative to alpha-hydroxy acids). Numerous clays can be blended to match your skin tone, or you can buy pre-mixed clay facials. _Clay is good for eliminating skin toxins and purifying pores_.

BODY MOISTURIZERS

The most of lotions and creams are water and oil emulsions. Any emulsion requires a preservative to avoid or destroy the aggregation at the interface between the oil and the water molecule of potentially dangerous bacteria. A high-quality natural emulsion should contain pressed natural cold and not processed oil or kinds of butter, and other nutritional substances such as aloe juice or gel, hydrosols, medicinal, and herbal water to name a few will be part of the water portion. It also uses only natural and organic preservatives such as grapes extract, meaning a product can last for three to six months. However, the quality of the drug is its freshness, and you should make sure that the cream is made in limited quantities.

Simple to read and comprehend ingredients. Pay attention to scientific or botanical names that use the traditional name for extracts and essential oils so that you can quickly recognize them in the future. Immediately after a heated bath or shower, the perfect way to use a moisturizer. After bath or shower the pores are open, and the oils are processed by the skin easier.

Another way is to wash the skin with hot wax.

Recipe: Melt two teaspoons (3 or 4 if you have more of your favorite butter(s) (shea, mango, or cacao) or if you have a friend with whom you can enjoy this special treat) in double-boiler. Apply 4-8 drops of essential oils, depending on the strength required. Should not overheat because heat will kill some of the oils' benefits. Massage oils on the whole body. The oils penetrate quickly, leaving the skin smooth and dry.

PERFUMES

Traditional art and perfumery technology have been revitalized. Many holistic shoppers have returned after decades of mass-produced, synthetic fragrances, overpriced, to the concept of wearing natural customized fragrances. Ensure sure you just use the natural resins or essential oils (e.g., *Vanilla oleoresin)* for your perfume. Natural fragrances are typically available as splashes, rolls on, or wax sticks, filled with fragrances that are rubbed into the skin.

MAKEUP

Natural cosmetics that do not contain talc, dyes, or additives are now available. Earth minerals are polished, while natural oils and botanicals are used for texture. The result is hypoallergenic and appealing.

How to Detox - Homemade Skin Care

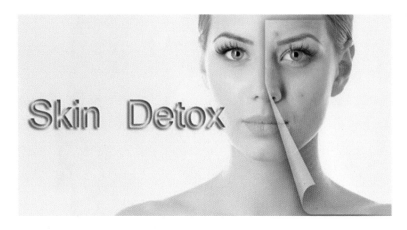

Learning how to detox will help you have the best possible results. ***What is detoxifying?*** This is a method of eliminating toxins and contaminants from the body in order to restore energy levels and to enhance optimal health. Our bodies are invaded every day by contaminants from a number of various causes, including factory gases, combustion emissions, pollution, cigarettes, alcohol, dietary additives, nicotine, prescription medications, noxious chemicals, obesity, tension, etc. Don't spend your resources on expensive vitamin powders, drinks, juices, or vitamins. You will detox with a quick change of diet and fast routines. ***Find simple ways to flawless detox skin at home!***

Adjust your bad eating habits!

ANTIOXIDANT FOODS

Avoid or at least reduce the daily intake of caffeine, refined sugar, saturated fats, coffee, and tobacco. Such chemical inhibitors will slow the Detox. Choose a good amount of antioxidant foods instead. Colorful fruit and vegetable foods contain high antioxidant amounts of vitamins A, C, E, and beta-carotene. The benefits of antioxidant-provided foods include potatoes, bananas, peas, onions, strawberries, snowflakes, green peppers, tomatoes, and broccoli. Even more antioxidant foods are available!

ANTIOXIDANT DRINKS

Stay away from high-sugar beverages. Search for 100% raw fruit juices or make your own organic juices freshly squeezed. Granite juice contains plenty of antioxidants. It's a very good drink from the heart! Many beverages include grape juice, blackberry juice, pomegranate juice, orange juice, apple juice, white tea, and green tea. It can be very helpful for people with busy lives to have an antioxidant drink in your everyday routine.

Drink tea to detox from the contaminants! The Mayo Clinic (https://www.mayoclinic.org)recommends the general law of "8 x 8." The skin consists of water-containing cells. When it has not provided the right amount of water, it can cause many skin disorders, such us redness, bad skin conditions: flaky, less durable, more vulnerable to wrinkling, wrinkles, flaws, and other. Do not be bothered, and this improved state is only transient as you seek to get rid of blackheads, blemishes or wrinkles, and note a weakening effect from drinking water. Over time the toxins have formed and are now washed out of the blood. Acne breakouts are smaller as the toxins are eliminated from the skin.

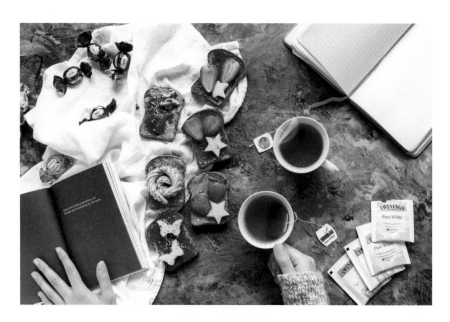

DETOX DIET!

Be vigilant if a "detox diet" is in place. ***Detox diets are not suitable for everyone!*** Weak or healthy adolescents with diabetes and heart failure or other medical problems, better pay attention! If you are pregnant or have an eating disorder, elimination diets should be stopped. Additives to Detox can have side effects. Many nutrients are fatigue, mineral imbalances, and digestion disorders caused by laxatives. Fasting will also contribute to a sluggish metabolic rate. Do not go on this without consulting the doctor.

Be wise. Seek for healthy, antioxidant, nutritional recettes. Check for detox diet cookbooks in your nearest bookstores. Such recipe books can also be downloaded online. If you read consumer reviews before you buy online, it could help you determine if a certain cookbook is better for you than another book.

DRY SKIN BRUSHING

The brushing of dry skin has been used for decades in the world. This gentle and productive procedure activates lymph channels and nerve endings, enhances blood supply, extracts dead cells, improves skin strength, enhances cell regeneration, reduces stubborn pores, and more! Dry brushing is an effective way to purify the lymph system. Skin rubbing promotes waste substance release from cells near the body's skin. Last but not least, certain toxins and their carrier cells make their way to the colon for disposal. Dry shaving of skin purifies the skin by extracting the cloak with calming acid. Skin can contract, decrease cellulite, and have an overall youthful, young look. As part of their routine, many beauty salons use dry brushing of skin.

Using an all-natural, non-synthetic brush with vegetable fiber. Broses of synthetic fiber can irritate the skin. Brushes are available in small or long styles of handles. Large handle bosses are more comfortable for areas like your back that can be difficult to touch. Hot brushes are to be used, fresh, but you can use wet brushes. Until your bath or shower, continuously rub the skin from the outside to the middle of your body in strokes. Start with the feet's soles. **ATTENTION!** Evite rashes, burns, bruises, fungi, poison oak, poison ivy, or skin patches that are damaged. Do not dry the hair, breast nipples, or sensitive body part. Using soft, gentle strokes across the breasts section.

Then take a hot shower or bath and a cold rinse to improve the circulation of the blood, then dry out well. You should then massage the skin with natural plant oils, including cocoa, almond, avocado, sesame, sunflower, or apricot oil. It all depends on your decision.

Clean your brush with soap and water at least once a week. When washing, try not to make wood too dirty. Wet wood can cause warping. Place your brush in a warm, free, sunny position to prevent mold and mildew growth.

Extended absorption time in hot water removes contaminants by swallowing and lymphatic draining. It promotes blood supply and facilitates the regeneration of skin cells. Detox at home with a steam bath, sauna, pool, or hot water bath! Bath salts can help to purify, exfoliate, and detoxify the skin. Normal salt pools, salts from the Dead Sea, goat's milk and MSM, are especially efficacious. MSM is a white crystal, natural, organic, non-toxic, odorless. It looks like a sugared surface. MSM is a strong element that detoxifies! MSM allows the free flow of water and nutrients into the cells when waste and toxins are released. MSM advantages from skincare include: minimizing swelling, decreasing chronic fatigue, relieving the muscle or joint pain, improving the body's heart tissue, detoxifying the bloodstream, increasing blood supply, minimizing the presence of aging, and helping to heal minor injuries.

Springing in a bath of natural bath salts allows an osmosis cycle to promote the exchange of contaminants in the body for the minerals required, which are dissolved in the water. Commercial or domestic bath salts may be scentless or aromatherapy-free.

Look for commercial or homemade facial cream with natural extracts including rosemary, cucumber, allantois, chamomile Romanesque and maize, and green tea!

FACE CREAM with GREEN TEA

Green tea, in fact, is a powerful antioxidant. This is anti-inflammatory and anti-bacterial. Skin rejuvenation, coloring, sun damage control, elasticity, shades, and protection. Most of us lead busy lives, but regular practice can: muscle tone, increasing oxygen and cell nutrients, reducing body contaminants, and optimizing digestion.

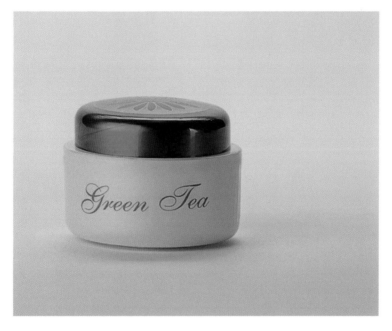

EXERCISE!

It is important that you do not put too much tension or a burden on your immune system. You must know how to keep pace. For starters, go exercising about thirty minutes a day, at least three days a week, with a good revitalizing pace while exercising.

The diaphragm, a muscle situated between a chest and a stomach cavity, induces deep breathing. It's different from breathing in the shallow or chest. Deep respiratory workouts are helpful in burning fat, stimulating metabolism, increasing energy, reducing stress, reducing anxiety, in reducing blood pressure, in strengthening abdominal and intestinal muscles. It enables endorphins to be produced in the body. The movement of the diaphragm up and down increases the blood flow and helps eliminate toxins.

Yoga exercise is a means of regulating deep breathing. This study of ancient India is renowned for its academic, physical, and spiritual observations. It is renowned for its cumulative, stimulating, therapeutic, and healing effect on the body. **_Face/facial yoga_**: A lot of us work out the muscles in our body, but we usually overlook the muscles in our face. And yet, we have tons of delicately intertwined facial muscles. It makes sense that they would merit their own workout session! That's where face yoga comes in!

What is Face Yoga and How Does It Tone Our Skin?

Face yoga is a series of specific movements that target, tone, and strengthen the facial muscles.

Glowing skin is a side effect of a good face workout!

Face yoga has a relaxing and regenerating effect on our skin. *"When we work our face muscles, we stimulate our facial pressure points, which promotes relaxation. A relaxed face always looks healthier and brighter than a tense one."*

Face yoga is a very good way to relax the muscles in your jaw, eyes, and head that become tense when you spend a lot of time in front of screens or on the phone, or if you have bad posture for other reasons. Working your facial muscles promotes better microcirculation and smoothes out wrinkles, giving your skin a healthy glow.

Face Yoga – 6 Exercices to Do at Home: Face yoga expert Danielle Collins made this video for Marie Claire Magazine UK

https://www.youtube.com/watch?time_continue=2&v=Vb_xcKcYs0Q&feature=emb_title

Be wise and clever when your body is detoxified. Choose products that are balanced, organic, and antioxidant. Be fully conscious of the industrial or homemade skincare items 'ingredients. Allow time to activate your body and push it! Relax now and then, and take a deep breath. Your body is built to cleanse itself already.

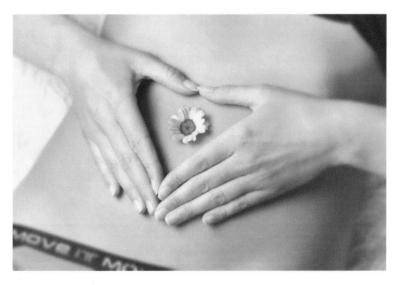

Natural Home Remedies For Sensational Spring Hair

What a wild winter we've had this year! It seems like year after year, the winters get colder and wetter. So it is wonderful news; finally, spring officially began, and we could be in for an unseasonably warm summer this year from some weather reports. So, let us keep our fingers crossed now for a good summer, but the spring has actually come for now, and you should try to keep your hair clean and gorgeous this spring here.

Trim Those Ends

Throughout the dreary cold, damp, and gloomy winter months, our hair was not really liked. It actually sat under a hat, or was covered in a blanket, or was usually only concealed. The cold, harsh winds have sucked life away, and hair can tend to break and incredibly harsh, particularly at the ends. Then it's time to book your favorite hairdresser and let them magically cut those dried and broken ends. Not only does that give the hair a new look and sound, but it also gives you the added bonus of a new attitude arriving in the spring.

Hair Mask

We all know we could put mud masks then hydrating masks on the bodies, but many of us do not know that by putting a mask on our hair, we can produce the same effects. From the winter hair can be seriously affected and separated from natural oils by the time we spend in chemically dried houses and workplaces. Now that spring has come, and we'll expose our hair to the world a lot more, let's bring back some of this moisture. Any beauty shop can buy a hair mask, but it is not only environmentally viable to make it natural from ingredients available around the house but also is even healthier than us since we can customize the hair mask to our own unique needs. An all-round formula for a perfect hair mask is a hair mask. ***Avocado oil can't beat as a natural beauty ingredient***. The oils in avocados are more like the natural oils of our hair and skin than the oils in prescription cosmetic goods obtained. Only pick up a few avocados and mash them until they're a simple paste. Add to wet, washed hair and leave for 15 minutes, wash with tepid water, leaving the hair silky and shiny.

Protein Treatments

We often watch movie stars on the red carpet and we think, "Oh, this person's hair is so thick and textured." The key to a body-full hair is protein. Protein hair treatments are trendy this season, and there are many items on the market that make such promises, but the most genuine protein hair treatment can be found right away in your cupboard. Egg yolks are made of protein, and natural oils and fats (e.g., Omega-3 fatty acids), these natural egg yolks content of our hair are used as beauty treatments.

Recipe: Take two egg yolks (battered) and add them to warm moist hair. Keep the egg for 20 minutes, then rinse it with cold water (make sure it's cold water and not hot!), then wash the face. The tremendous deal of protein and natural fats in the egg yolk will fill the hair with moisture and muscle, which have been lost in the cold season.

Remove Chlorine from Shower Water

No matter how many wraps, oils, or conditioners we place in our hair, there is one important part of our hair care regimen, which can do little if we do not deal with it. As we wash every day, we subject our hair to a water source saturated with chlorine. Chlorine is a particularly corrosive disinfectant used as a solvent in many industries.

Since making contact with some form of oils (whether these be the natural oils created by our bodies or the oils that we use in our hair treatments), it would automatically extract the oil. We need to take every care that we remove the chlorine in our showers until it reaches our bodies, and we can add a clear shower filter or a shower head with a filter in it. By extracting this chlorine, our hair will also contain natural oils that keep hair clean and beautiful, and if we do so with the above natural treatments, we are confident that our hair looks healthier during this spring than ever before.

UV Protecting Shampoo

Key recommendation for this spring is to use high-quality UV shampoo. UV safety shampoo Keep our fingers crossed; hopefully, this spring, we get a lot of sunlight. Even if we enjoy the hot rays of the sun and the lifting of our mood, the sun is shocking too in the form of toxic ultraviolet rays that can kill hair prematurely. Finding a UV shampoo of high quality from our nearest cosmetics shop is a must to protect hair from drying and aging effects of sunlight. While these natural treatments are an added bonus by maintaining the natural oils provided by our scalp, they do have a natural capacity to protect against UV radiation. Isn't Nature Mother great?

I hope you liked these little natural tips on the way to keep your hair clean and creative this spring and note that you are getting what you are putting in in terms of your wellbeing. Seek to raise our lives on pesticides and additives and strive to live more naturally.

Chamomile Tea Benefits - Homemade Skin Care and More!

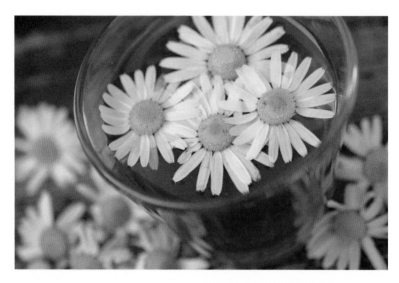

For decades, Chamomile tea advantages have been known. Chamomile looks like a daisy with white petals and gold discs. Throughout the early to mid-summer months, the flowers have a good fragrance and bloom. This is located near rivers, landfills or agricultural fields in Europe, Asia, North America, and Australia. The name is also known as Wild Chamomile, Hungarian Chamomile, and Pineapple Herb.

The word "chamomile" comes from Greek and means "earth-apple on the table." This is known for the sweet, apple-like fragrance of the herb. Chamomile tea is a sweet, fruity, and golden shade.

There are two species that come under the name of chamomile: Matricaria recutita and Chamaemelum Nobile. German chamomile is an annual herb and seasonal Roman chamomile.

They come from different chamomile plant types but look very similar and are used to handle similar situations interchangeably.

HEALTH BENEFITS & USES: *Skin Care*

Chamomile / Chamomile Tea Medicinal, Aromatherapy, Hair Care, Animal Care

MEDICINAL

There can be other health benefits of Tea! Chamomile is anti-viral, dietary, anti-microbial, antispasmodic, and anti-inflammatory. It alleviates: stomach upset, bowel disease irritable, heartburn, menstrual cramps, muscle spasm, back pain, arthritis rheumatoid, migraines, hypertension, sinus infections, toothache, insomnia, etc. Chamomile tea is abundant in Quentin, a coloring herb for fruits and vegetables. It tackles harm from free radicals. Glycine, a chamomile amino acid, helps keep the nervous system healthy. The chamomile tea will relax the nerves, alleviate tension and depression with a touch of lemon grass. Drink Herbal Tea before bed and battle insomnia. This drink is free of caffeine and is soothing, fruity, and sweet.

SKIN CARE

Chamomile improves recovery of superficial cuts, prevents skin damage from free radicals, (wrinkles, fine lines), slims up the skin tone, soothes wounds, soothes the scalp, (hives, stings of the bees, acne), removes the dark area under the eyes, and decreases inflammation and puffiness under the eyes, and is useful to make the scalp healthy. This has highly effective skin treatment, purification, and antioxidant properties that have been shown to help suppress acne and acne rash. This helps eliminate blackheads and tends to reduce acne. Chamomile alleviates skin infections, teeth, and gums removed. This is used for mouth washing or gargling. Chamomile tea, combined with powdered milk, is an exfoliating skin paste. To minimize puffiness, put under eyes cooled chamomile tea bags. Essential Blue Chamomile and Roman chamomile oils also have skin-soothing powers. Blue basic chamomile oil has a high concentration of blue azulene with a blue tint. This chamomile comes from the German chamomile vine. Any Blue chamomile was only grown for medicines. Chamomile is used for the consumer and handmade products, soaps, skin creams, lotions, facial, and other uses!

For a natural home-made facial cream, a roman chamomile extract may be combined with other natural ingredients, including aloe Vera, rosemary, and cucumber. This will have smooth, soft skin filled with natural, hydrating, balanced nutrients. Chamomile can be used to produce organic soap. Mixed with oils mixed with soap, chamomile will help to cure home-induced acne and relax dry, itchy skin.

HAIR CARE

Chamomile is widely used as a blond hair care product. It slowly lightens and lightens hair as used as a rinse. It adds golden highlights to the constant brown hair. You will use chamomile in industrial or handmade shampoos. It improves the hair and helps to heal split ends. It helps to avoid dry and oily scalp conditions.

Roman and Moroccan natural chamomile oils are used for aromatherapy purposes. Moroccan chamomile is not a real plant of chamomile. This is commonly used in perfume mixtures and in aromatherapy. Roman basic chamomile oil is used in skin care products and aromatherapy for its skin-soothing properties. Calm nerves even by inhaling fresh or dried chamomile.

FACTS

About one million cups of chamomile tea are drunk each year. It is a popular tea for medical, nutritional, skin care, hair treatment, pet care, and everyday enjoyment. Tea and blends are sold in convenience shops, pharmacies, organic food outlets, retail, and elsewhere. There are many benefits of chamomile tea, but there are always precautions.

ATTENTION! Chamomile or chamomile Tea may have side effects. Such as: low risks of diarrhea Allergic Skin Reactions: hives, fever, itching Allergic skin Reactions: tightness in the arms, swelling in the neck, mouth, ears, lips or tongue, rabies, menstrual changes. Avoid use when breastfeeding. Prevent using when on blood thinners. Prevent use if allergic to ragweed!

CHAPTER FOUR

10 Myths About Hair

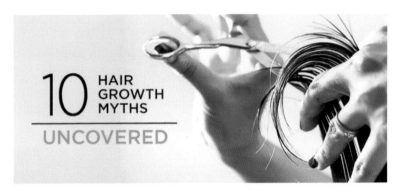

**Here are the top ten beauty misconceptions, and why the perfect locks aren't useful.**

**10) Anxiety contributes to hair loss.**

It can be so because you have recently endured traumatic experience like divorce or some tragic accident. The hair could fall, but it will return. The average human loses nearly 100 strands of natural shedding per day. Sometimes, I lose so much hair daily, but I have no problems with my health or hormones. It happens to appear some period like this, depends of which season is.

However, if you experience a serious hair loss, you can consult with your GP.

**9) Don't pluck grey hair-two when rising in place.** When a gray hair strand appears, the hair strand will stay gray (unless you color it).

8) Ice water makes hair more shine.

I was also told to clean hair with cold water. You think it covers your hair follicle, but you don't know that it's just a way to wake up in the morning!

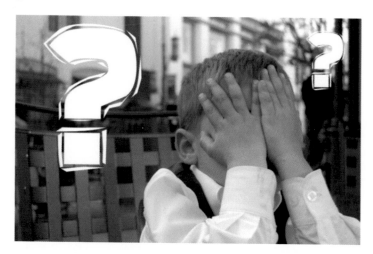

In fact, if you want shinier hair, use a cold air blast from your blow dryer according to your style. That locks in elegance and allows for more shine.

Then the next ...

7) 100 strokes a day!

Many of us have learned this myth: 100 strokes for good, lovely hair. It's so far from the truth that it's not funny! Hairbrushes will smash your hair and make it more damage then help.

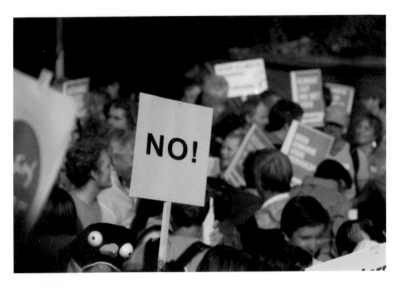

6) Use a nickel-size amount of conditioner.

I still wonder why a nickel-sized for the hair?

The truth is, if you have longer hair, you need more. You will feel the softness of your hair after applying the conditioner. My hair is extremely long, so I use about half a buck a day. This makes my hair soft; my hair would feel dry if I don't use as many. So, it just depends of the length of your hair.

5) Split ends may be "covered" by goods.

Now it's just crazy. Hair is dead cells; when a split ends happen, the hair shaft separates the middle. If not treated, the hair will start falling and, much worse, it will damage the scalp. These split ends have to be "sealed" by goods, but come on.

Consider your nails: if you break, what is going to fix it? Cutting it. Chopping it. Any glue may be added, but it often cracks and does further damage. Just trim it regularly so that your hair stays healthy.

4) Dandruff is caused by dry scalp.

Dandruff actually comes from oily hair, not dry scalp! They are two different ailments! If you have oily hair, use an anti-dandruff shampoo to get it nice and clean; if you have dry scalp, it is possible that you have some skin issue, in that case it is better to consult your dermatologist.

3) Hair products damage hair.

"Don't straighten your hair, or you'll damage it." "Don't dye it, or you'll dry it out."

Yadda It's 2020, people. Hair products are created for women who style their hair. Using the right products, you can protect your hair from further damage.

In fact, you're likely to find a lighter, shinier texture every time you dye your hair. There are so many vitamins and other coloring ingredients that your hair can benefit from.

Using a heat shield for extreme styling approaches (ex. straightening).

2) "Lather, rinse, repeat." This is something we learn so much that it has become commonplace. You don't have to wash your hair twice to make your shampoo work, I repeat. A shampoo will do the "job" even with one wash (if you are using the right shampoo).

Once I had a case when a hairstylist "recommended" me to do that: I had a Brazilian Blowout, the double-shampoo exposed hair follicles to the keratin oil.

1) Like hair longer? Trim it!

The only benefit of a regular trim is to get rid of split ends and to keep your hair shape. Hair doesn't grow evenly around your head, so trimming keeps the ends at the same length, instead of one-sided.

Well, there you have it! Ten most common myths about hair, and the honest truth about them.

Maintain Youthful, Healthy and Beautiful Skin

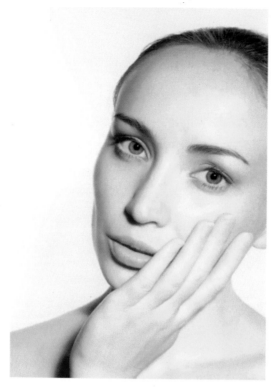

Individuals likewise have propensities like smoking, unhealthy eating regimen, and drinking, which plays a factor in deciding how old their skin will resemble. If you have mature skin and need to care for it appropriately, at that point two things ought to be on your list - _replenishing and safeguarding the moisture of the skin_. When that is done, different signs of aging like dullness, wrinkles, and lack of hydration; will be anything but difficult to manage. There are a few steps you need entirely to follow to accomplish these two objectives. Don't go out in the sun except if you need to. When you do, don't forget to put on your sun cream first. Select one that has an SPF factor of at least 30. Additionally, try to avoid sun exposure from the time between 10 a.m. also, 3 p.m. at the point when the sun is the strongest; if that is unavoidable, wear a hat.

If you see dark colored spots or any part of your skin, don't forget to consult your specialist or dermatologist. In the most cases is nothing to worry about but it is better to be safe and sound!

While treating your mature skin, go for products that don't have any siding agents, and that are without synthetic and non-liquor based. You can generously use products like petrolatum and lanolin. **Natural products like night primrose rose hips oils, pomegranate seed, and avocado are additionally extraordinary decisions**.

Utilizing mellow cleansers for cleaning and taking fewer baths will assist you with protecting your mature skin. Don't use high temp water while taking a shower as that evaporates skin; instead, absorb yourself warm water. After your bath, make sure to apply a decent lotion on the wet skin to capture the moisture of your skin.

To hinder the signs of aging, you need to recharge the moisture content of your skin routinely. For that, select a cream that has anti-oxidants and which will repair your skin. In any case, make sure to keep it basic; don't use various products or use it in exorbitant sum as that can further aggravate and damage your skin.

There are skin cells that don't shed effectively. To remove them, you need to use an exfoliant. Shedding routinely will remove a wide range of subtle skin pieces just as dead skin cells which are the purpose behind the harshness and dullness of your skin. After you shed, moisture can without much of a stretch feed your skin.

Aside from keeping up a skin care regime, you need to fortify yourself with right nourishment to recover that shine to your mature skin. For that, make beyond any doubt that you're eating regimen is wealthy in sustenance's with a high measure of nutrients, minerals, and omega 3 unsaturated fats. This works just as collagen of your skin. These nutrients are available in natural vegetable and organic products.

Saturating your skin must be done from inside also. So make beyond any doubt you drink in any event eight to ten glasses of water each day. Forgo taking juiced drinks and carbonated drinks. Instead, attempt green tea which may have caffeine; yet, besides, have such a significant number of other useful things that it is incredible for your wellbeing.

Tips For Oily Skin

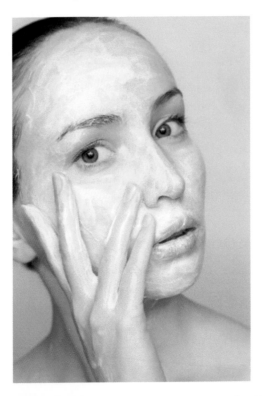

Oily skin is frequently the most difficult to manage. Oily skin is a problem that has provoked the skincare industry to make products intended to help combat the problem.

The problem isn't in finding products for this skin type, it is rather in discovering ones that work as promoted. To more readily comprehend this problem let begin by portraying it.

Oil production in the skin is natural and is the consequence of the sebaceous glands situated in the middle layer of skin called the dermis. These natural oils are expected to keep skin clammy and supple. Notwithstanding, for specific individuals, these sebaceous glands produce a lot of oil producing a skin type ordered mostly as oily skin.

First thing after waking to verify whether your skin has a shiny sheen to it, particularly at the point between your eyes or vertically down along your nose right to your jawline. If you have a bright polish on this piece of your face at that point, chances are high you have oily skin.

Oily skin is reaction by glands that produce more oil than normal. Notwithstanding trouble for your complexion, these oils are significant because they go about as the skin's natural moisturizer. The primary enticement is to begin evacuating all the oil. However, the better course is to monitor it by purging with warm water and a delicate gel cleanser.

When searching for oily skincare products, avoid oil-based products. Ensure the beautifying agents and sun protection you use are without oil. It looks terrible to add oil to skin that is as of now experiencing more oil than usual.

Second problem, oily skin is, at times, delicate. You can use oily skincare products with the label 'non-comedogenic' or 'non-acnegenic' on the names. Continuously recall that any oily skin care therapy ought to incorporate more than what you put on your skin.

To try to solve the problem, combine the elements of your skincare products carefully with appropriate skin care therapy.

Four Easy Steps to Keep your Hair Healthy

Bonus Summer Hair Care

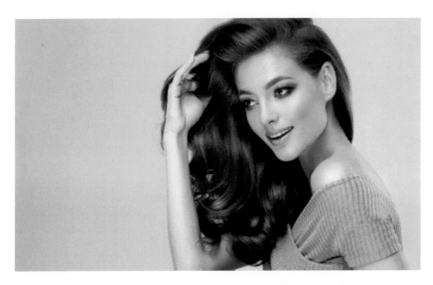

Through following the fast tips below, you can easily keep your hair healthy;

#1. Lead a balanced diet, we hear that all the time, but the truth about your hair is so, and that's why. The thin glans attached to your follicle (the base of your hair) contain a slick, oil-like material known as sebum. We are supposed to lubricate our hair and skin in order to keep it soft. Sebum contains fatty acids, cholesterol, and triglycerides from you and the body's nutrients. So, where do the body's foods come from? the food we're consuming. There is a very easy rule for good health. Superfoods. Superfoods are simply foods that contain two or three nutrients at exceptionally high amounts. Several examples are soybeans, walnuts, quinoa, acai, blueberries, oats, broccoli, and green tea. You will guard against cancer, premature aging, and reduced fitness. And of course, that will prevent your skin and hair from all the reserves of nutrients in your sebum sparkling with good protection.

#2. _Shampoo Less_ - Sure, but for many, like me, it's a difficult one. And for all of you who have struggled and eventually succeeded, tell the rest, how it really helped your hair.

#3. _Keep daily beauty appointments_ - When your hair is clean, and you want to preserve your style, go for trimming every four to six weeks. Because of the ends which split and fall, you just need two inches to be cut off. You want the hair to grow, but the ends do not grow as they fall up, and the hair can remain as it is or get shorter over time.

#4. _Mask once a week_ – Use conditioner any time you wash your hair. If you have an oily scalp, add it to the middle shaft at the ends. The difference between a mask and the packaging is like normal food in contrast with superfoods. It has added nutrients and is, therefore, denser and harder. Using both, is like feeding a number of vitamins to your hair, so you never get used to a collection of ingredients. For a while, we have been using our beloved conditioner, and then it just seems to stop running at some point. The explanation is that the hair is fresh and needs new nutrients. But the same thing persists over time as you turn to the new product. So you can try new products and see how your hair will respond to it. But always pay attention on ingredients.

Summer Hair Care – Mission Impossible?

The question we ask ourselves every August as we run our fingers through our sun and salt water soaked ends of hair is: How do you nourish your hair when everything in the summer I expose to, is actually harmful to it?

Summer sun, high temperatures and salt water can really do a lot of damage to our hair. Although each of us wants a beach waves hairstyle, and gorgeous beach hair, most of us head straight for the hairdresser after the summer because of the dry areas and the hair.

Both during the winter and in the summer, hair care needs to be enhanced. What needs to be done to preserve the shine and health of your hair during the summer?

- *__Avoid dryer, straightener, and curler!__*

That's one of the tips with a big exclamation mark! Of course, I need not tell you that hair straighteners are not good for the care of your hair, because you already know it, but we are here to remind you that a natural look is really the best and healthiest solution.

- *__Avoid products with strong chemical ingredients__*

Your hair is exposed to high temperatures and UV rays all summer long. Try to strike a balance by using as mild as possible products that do not contain too many chemicals to preserve her health as much as possible.

- *__In fact, you don't need shampoo on a daily basis__*

If you are on vacation, and you come to your room every day at a resort with hair drained and salted from seawater, you don't always have to use shampoo to wash off the salt. Rinse it well, then apply some balm to the ends, wait a while, then rinse again... And voilà, the hair is fresh and shiny again!

- *__Use hair products with a protective factor__*

There are many natural hair care products with a protective factor, such as macadamia oil, that are used without flushing. Always have one in your beach bag, as he will be your best ally when it comes to summer hair care!

And finally, the best advice on how to care for your hair is one that no brand, or even your hairstylist will tell you - take care of yourself. A healthy body can be recognized by hair, skin, and nails. Vitamins, proteins, and hydration are what your body and even your hair need. Hairstyle, color, and length of hair are a matter of taste, but the health of your hair is solely down to the care and care you will give it.

CHAPTER FIVE

Natural Hair Color

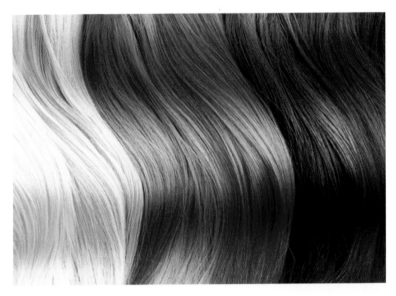

Naturally, 'dye' the hair, without additives, no paint, no fake dyes. Commercially available Hair Coloring uses chemicals to replace, substitute, or improve the natural hair shaft pigments. There are other adverse consequences that can be caused by their use;

Skin scratching, pain, swelling, inflammation, redness, discomfort-chemicals such as PPD (p-Phenylenediamine) allergies-hair breakage or fading, over-processing-colors of the skin or drying-coloring unpredicted (mostly in the home) and adverse effects mentioned above are more severe issues regarding safety and possible chemical hazards. Although some debate is taking place on the nature of hair coloring issues, the chance actually does not have to be taken.

<u>Publications on the hazards of hair dyes are available, including:</u>

- An FDA report that found lead acetate to be harmful in several colors.

- Papers relating to the production of some types of cancer, including leukemia, non-Hodgkin's lymphoma, lung cancer, multiple myeloma caused by hair dye use.

- Repeated use of permanent dark hair coloration can theoretically double the chance of a person having different types of blood cancer.

- Many scientists believe hair bleach can destroy cells in the brain.

- Many home hair dyes found a known human carcinogen, 4-ABP.

<u>Natural hair colors like plant powders Henna, Indigo, Cassia, and Amla can be used easily to improve or alter your hair's color.</u> These are herb powders combined with water, lemon juice, and yogurt in your own home to make a paste on your face and hair.

Since they don't knock the normal pigment out of your scalp, their appearance will depend on the appearance of your scalp. For example, henna used solely on white hair produces red, while straight henna on brown hair produces auburn hair.

Such powders can also be used securely on chemically conditioned or teased hair. You should use them comfortably as much as you like. You will quickly intensify your hair with another treatment if you paint with these powders, and you have a hue that is not dark enough.

The final color of the shampoo takes a few days, as it will start to remain in the hair shaft for a few days because of the oxidation cycle. This natural cycle happens as plant dyes are equally exposed to the sun, as a cut apple is brown over time.

You would definitely note that most hairdressers are 'anti-henna' because they are just treated to 'composite' hennas, combined with dyes, acetate plastic, or other metal fasteners.

Check for allergic reactions, as for any products. You should always try pasta on a little amount of hair (take hair out of your hairbrush) and see what color your hair should get.

HOW TO USE THESE NATURAL COLORANTS

You don't have to premix the powder with lemon juice, whether you are using Amla or Indigo.

Only HENNA or CASSIA NEED TO BE MIXED WITH LEMON JUICE AND Stay OVERNIGHT.

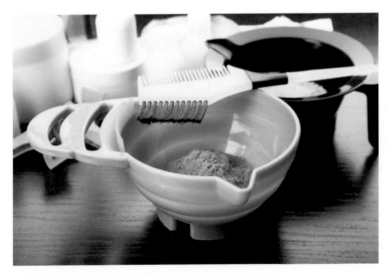

Henna powder

Henna may be blended with Indigo and Amla, until ready to submit.

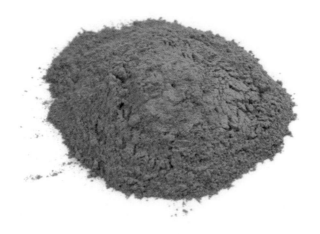

Cassia powder

Regardless which powder mix you use, follow these rules for mixing: 100 g of powders for short hair, 200 g for neck length, long hair straight hair, 300 g for shoulder-length, straight hair back, 500 g for tail end straight hair.

Mix henna or cassia with enough lemon juice to create a mashed potato paste. Using orange juice, grapefruit juice, or less acidic liquid than citrus juice if the skin becomes lemon reactive and itchy after using henna.

Fill the paste bottle with plastic wrap and let it sit at room temperature or moist surroundings overnight. The acid in the citrus juice extracts the color from the plant material, as henna or cassia rest. This gradual, acidic release is the best outcome for you. Once the pasta is finished, add a little more lemon juice or tea to make the paste as smooth as yogurt. Apply a little at a time to achieve the required consistency.

For Indigo or Amla, simply blend the consistency of yogurt with ample water to paste. Lemon juice is not required. Only use warm water and apply a little to it at a time so that it is not too dry. When your Indigo or Amla are blended, all the pasta you want to blend can be combined. And make sure that you swirl it so that you don't have hair streaked.

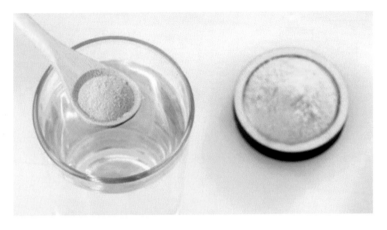

Amla powder

You can also first add a paste, let it hang, rinse it, and then place another paste on your hair. You can get a lighter or brighter color if you add the pastes separately.

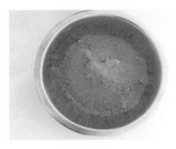

Indigo powder

For beginning, you should first color your hair with henna, then color it with indigo after your henna has dried. You can only blend henna and indigo together and add as a single piece if you don't want as dark a black.

This method can get sticky, so wear gloves! You should prepare smaller quantities in full colors to protect the roots. Health studies indicate the henna relaxes and can relieve headaches. When you have a lot of hair, the paste will feel heavy on your skin.

To add the paste to your hair, wash and dry your hair, then peel. For simpler use, you may want to split your hair. Start from the back and work the paste across the hair. Apply the paste-like frosting thickly. More henna makes the stain darker and stronger. Put the next segment down to close the next segment.

Repeat until all your hair is covered, and then gather up all your hair and tie in plastic tape. If you want to cover with an old towel, but if the paste gets on the towel, it can become colored. After dying, clean any visible traces.

The paste need to stay 2-4 hours on your hair before you test the color. Meanwhile, you can find a quiet spot and relax.

Finally, wash your hair with the shampoo, as regular and dry.

The hair can have a scent for a few days. When you do not like the paste/powder scent, cook a tablespoon of lavender bud or rosemary powder in water, squeeze the rest of the plant and rinse your hair with rosemary or lavender tea to combat the herbicide scent. Or, before you apply, you might add cinnamon to the paste.

At first, henna-fared hair can look too bright in color but don't panic! That will darken for the next two days. Then you will see the hair true color.

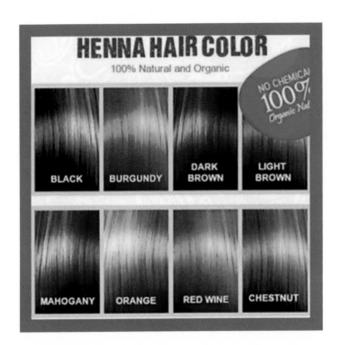

Indigo can generate a wide variety of colors when used in Henna or alma, resulting in dark colors from natural dark brunette or black hair colors. Unlike Henna, it is a clear paste or alkaline, and it does not require lemon juice to enable it.

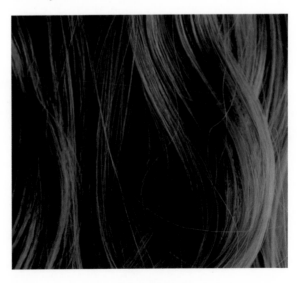

Indigo black

Amla makes a lighter brown using Henna and Indigo. Amla is possibly the finest hair conditioner in existence. You can use the paste regularly to cover, clean, and make your hair shine. Amla can be used to strengthens waves and curves. Also you can use Amla to treat grey hair.

Cassia is an outstanding conditioner for hair, independent of the color. Cassia is a green leaf powder which, mixed with water, tastes like mown grass. This is alkaline like Indigo and does not have to activate the color molecule by lemon juice. It gives golden tones for blonde or grey hair. You can blend it with some other powder mixture or alone.

The conditioning results last roughly one month. You can mix cassia or henna in brown, strawberry brown, and copper red colors.

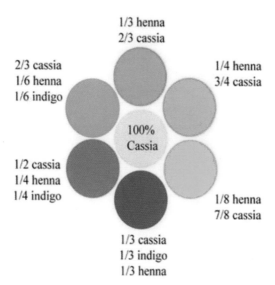

The Truth About Silicones and Their Effect on Natural Hair

Each woman decide whether the use of silicones is worth the cost or not. And how much is it a risk? I've found that some people find like the reward by using it. Nonetheless, those who take the gamble to use silicone-based goods have made well-informed decisions.

Silicone vs Natural Hair

Silicones were dressed as mates with natural hair. They are here to help fight hair abuse and to ease some of the burdens we put on us. However, we discover later that the use of silicones just prolongs the inevitable and can make matters worse. One of the disappointments of silicones is that they can absorb humidity and act as a humectant. Dry hair requires humidity, right?

The main trouble with silicones is that they are not water-soluble, which means that they can accumulate in the hair over time, and they are very hard to get rid of. We need to use very strong sulfates (shampoos) to get out of this mess and get out of this build-up. It has been discovered that shampoos containing these sulfates are not safe for us, because they rob our hair of everything possible to protect its health.

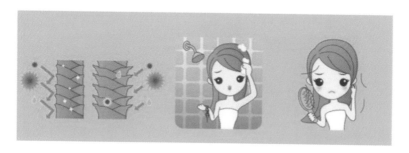

I am also not entirely sure what long-term harm silicones can do, but an uneducated hypothesis would be that the continued use of silicones could exacerbate the long-term damage by using rough goods. Another factor to remember that if silicones are effective at capturing stuff like heat, then I'll say they can also capture impurities, and this may also arise when the problems happen.

It is all too bad because silicones make it much harder to find ways to suit our natural tresses. True, silicones are a quick remedy. I'm searching for more natural hair solutions that can give me comparable results as silicones, but this isn't easy ...

Still... Maybe there's hope!

I found that some silicones may be appropriate for us naturalists. When the silicone is mentioned in front of the nasty cone with a term, *Polyethylene Glycol (PEG),* then it can be helpful on natural hair. PEG is a water-soluble silicone that does not build up the drug. Many of those that use shampoos or co-wash our hair with the conditioners are in a position to keep our hair clean and moisturized with certain ingredients or processes.

There are moments when life calls for what fits right now, I agree. I know that at times it takes a bit longer than you can expect to invest at your best. There are silicone-free items out there that moisturize the hair. You just have to work and figure out what these things are.

This is for the purpose of knowledge only. Like always, ensure that you do the homework to select the right things for your beauty. I send this knowledge to people interested in using natural foods that do not have time or will actually purchase their goods instead of making them themselves.

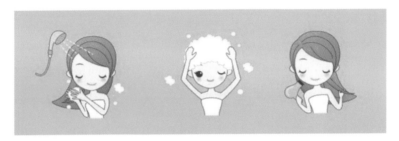

The Advantage of Balmain Hair Extensions

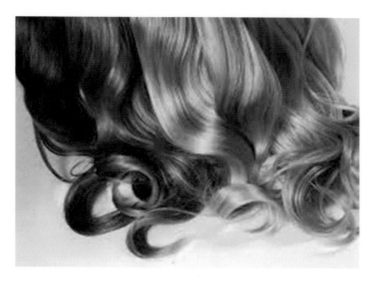

Hair extension is a common addition to hair of modelers, television stars, and women who work in the public eye. It is used by thousands of people every day. Any woman who wishes to add texture to her locks now has the possibility of creating items such as Balmain hair extensions.

Balmain's hair extension (https://store.balmainhair.com/nl/?store=dutch) dealer is based in the Netherlands. It is renowned all over the world for making outstanding beauty products. The demand for their outstanding hair enhancement offerings is increasing today. In such goods, only human hair is used, which means that whether you have single or double styles, it can be handled the same as your own production.

There is also a clip-on design available. This one can be put on and brought anywhere. It is always a great way to illustrate a particular hue. It is surprising that a woman with a different color string on her head represents the hue of the robe. Teenagers who choose a beautiful orange, red, green, or another hue that is easily visible always want this.

The clip-ons are available in various designs. You may choose a gap, a ponytail, or something that has been used in the public eye. It enables a person to quickly alter his entire look. Picture going to school or at a special event where the development becomes limp and unexpectedly sumptuous or when stylish bangs emerge on one's face.

Having this form of extension is, in many ways, useful for people who want the most favorable view of their hair. People with slim growth consider that gives them a lovely appearance that looks normal and absolute on their heads. Nobody can claim it's not a part of one's natural development.

Both external characteristics are straight or curved, short, or long. In addition, colors may be applied to suit or state your natural keys. These colors, without destroying your own growth, can be added or removed at will.

If you're not pleased with your hair's present state, you can make a full improvement that is beautiful when extensions are attached. This is a shame that some women are rising thinly on their hands. It may be attributed to an inherited trait or a disorder. It is a way of having a normal and full-fledged appearance, which can only be used when added to the eyes.

These styles of hair tips have long been around, and a nylon formula commonly used does not have the same feel as natural production. Fortunately, the human hair used today has structure and blends well with natural development. Balmain hair extensions have a six months warranty for their items, and most orders include a special shampoo, packaging, and care.

The present use of hair extensions has improved significantly with the introduction of brands such as Balmain hair extensions. These have been used for years by celebrities, film stars, and well-known figures, and are now open to the general public. It is a great way to add texture or totally change your hairstyle.

The selection of colors and patterns is incredible. They are straight or curved, long or short, and can perfectly suit your natural development. Therefore, colors can be inserted or removed without injury. One's look may be changed drastically for every reason or even for everyday wear.

You will change the appearance of your hair absolutely with these kinds of adds. It can be changed from short to long, straight to curved, and other variations for an entirely new feel. This is particularly true of women with a slender growth that can look whole-hearted and ordinary.

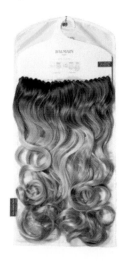

Balmain Hair Extension

Blemish-Prone Skin

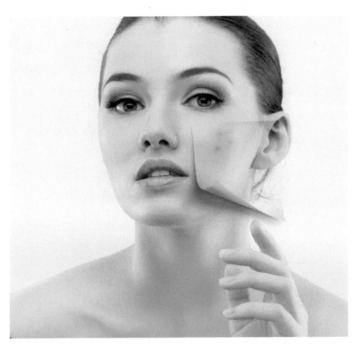

The most of people have problem of blemish-prone skin. Or on the other hand, as dermatologists call it - *ACNE*. Dermatologist are revealing as much as 70% of their patients presently are seeking help with their steady blemishes.

Blemished skin can significantly influence our social and expert lives. It can make us pull back from others, keep distance from connections, and keep down on seeking that next activity advancement. Complete confidence can be folded over our powerlessness to control how our skin looks. Grown-up endures are paying attention to this problem tremendously.

For most blemish sufferers, be that as it may, the news is high. Although there is no remedy for acne, we CAN securely control and manage the breakouts. Furthermore, you DO need to manage and control them - else you'll experience post-acne inconveniences, for example, staining of the skin (dark colored spots from past blemishes) and to top it all off - scarring.

Medicines for acne have significantly advanced throughout the years. Brilliant science reveals that if you treat your whole face, reliably every morning and consistently, with the right formulations, you can manage most blemish-prone skin problems. The formulations must contain just *non-comedogenic ingredients*. A blemish is essentially a clogged pore, so we can't utilize ingredients that clog the pores on our skin. Products should first - quiet the skin's aggravations (botanicals like chamomile and aloe are the best), also - unclog the pores and dispose of the fitting of oil and microscopic organisms, and third - tenderly shed the skin to expel dead skin that can clog the pores.

Now and then all you need is a daily schedule of two times a multi-day utilizing naturally based skin care products to get the ideal outcomes. However, if despite everything you're breaking out, you should take a stab at using organically based products that likewise contain over the counter strength medicines, for example, *sulfur, benzoyl peroxide, and alpha hydroxy acids.* If, following a little while on this regimen, despite everything you don't have your blemishes leveled out, it is suggested that you see a dermatologist quickly for medicine strength medicated skin care products to get your acne leveled out. The significant thing is - don't pause! The condition will decline, and now you'll manage the complexities also.

As a rule, you may need to utilize the medicated products for a brief timeframe, until your skin is cleared, and afterward, you can bite by bit change your regimen back to absolutely natural. If you discover your skin erupting once more, you can backpedal on the medicated products as needed.

If you're one of the millions battling with blemish-prone skin, know, you're not the only one. Numerous others are experiencing the same battles from you. There is trust! I urge you to act today, look for exhortation from a skin care proficient. Approach them for their proposals for a twice everyday skin care regimen that treats the whole skin, is organically based, with non-comedogenic ingredients, contains over the counter medications (if needed), tenderly peels, quiets the skin, unclogs pores and battles microscopic organisms.

CHAPTER SIX

How to Detox - Homemade Skin Care Recipes

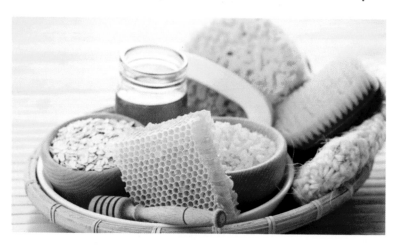

Learn how to detox you skin at home!

Nowadays on internet you can find a bunch of Homemade Skin Care Recipes, but not quite all really works for everybody. When experimenting with your at home ingredients, you should be careful, because if it happens that you have been allergic on some ingredient you can have more "problems" on your skin than benefits.

12 recipes for your homemade face scrub

Do you regularly use face scrub or you skip this form of care? learn How to make Homemade face scrub and why it is necessary for facial care!

Each of us has a different approach to cleaning our face. There are women who regularly nourish their face and take care of every detail and make sure to use a face scrub. On the other side, there are women who don't even know how useful a face scrub is. Oh yes, there are some women who will go to bed with makeup on without a bit of conscience.

If you are one of those women who skips this type of care, this text is like made for you! Find out what you missing, and how easy it is to make a homemade face scrub!

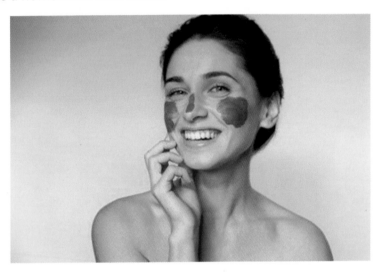

Benefits!

If you have ever asked advice on how to make your facial skin beautiful, how to get rid of acne, and how to properly nourish your skin or get rid of your wrinkles you will find that regular face scrub is a step you should not skip.

You may be among those who think that the tiny particles in these facial treatments are damaging and scratching the skin and that this is not an option for sensitive facial skin. The truth is that you need to make good choices when it comes to ingredients, and the natural ones are definitely the best!

Why it is a necessary step in skin care?

Because it helps your skin recover faster. New skin cells are created in the inner layer of the skin called the dermis. On this occasion, old skin cells are expelled - to a part of the skin known as the epidermis and they gradually fall off from the face, if you allow them.

If you do not properly nourish the face, or you do not clean it properly, but therefore regularly you apply on it a ton of cream or makeup, these cells do not fall off your face but rather find their place in your pores. When the pores get stuck, pimples will come out.

Fine particles in face scrub remove dead skin cells, stimulate surface circulation and make skin smoother, healthier and super toned. Not only that, but the skin that is released from dead cells better absorbs all those ingredients that you apply with creams or masks against wrinkles or pimples.

If you have dry skin that is dandruff, regular face scrub will help remove dead cells from the skin and make it look smooth again!

How to use face scrub properly?

You should know how often you can use this type of skin care and whether you will overdo if you do it every day.

Everyday facial scrub is too much. 2-3 times a week is enough if you have oily skin and once a week if your skin is dry.

Also, not every treatment is good for every skin type. That is why when making a natural face scrub you need to choose the right ingredients accordingly. First, consider what natural ingredients you will use as an abrasive to remove dead cells.

Mostly used are sugar, coffee, baking soda, salt, corn flour.

Salt has very hard particles and can damage the skin so it is not for those with sensitive skin that is prone to irritation, but is full of minerals, especially with sea salt. Sugar scales less, but make sure it is not too bulky. It is excellent because it is a natural source of glycolic acid that is fantastic for skin care.

After this step, you should choose the base for these abrasive particles that suits you the best.

Most often these are some natural oils that are good for the face. Olive oil, almond oil, coconut oil are just some of which you can use to make a natural face scrub. They are not heavy and very oily and will help keep the skin hydrated, soft and supple after treatment.

Lastly, choose an ingredient that will add vitamins and minerals and nourish your skin.

In other words, since we are talking about natural variants, some herbal supplement, fruits or vegetables, cereals or honey. What you add depends on the problem you are treating. Strawberries are full of Vitamin C and lighten the skin, great against the scars on the face. Pineapple is good against pimples, oats soften the skin.

Facial scrubs are not for everyone. If you have very sensitive skin and skin problems, warts, wounds, eczema herpes and similar changes, this is not the treatment for you.

You can apply this treatment on your face, but you must avoid the eye area. Take my word for it, not only is this skin part delicate and sensitive, but some of the ingredients become itchy and painful when they come in contact with the eyes.

Make a face scrub by yourself

It's not hard to make a natural face scrub, and it's not too expensive either. Just keep in mind that you are not making too much, because natural ingredients do not contain preservatives and such mixtures become bad relatively quickly if you do not use them immediately.

Any excess left over can be stored in the refrigerator for up to max. three days.

Here are some quick and easy recipes to try:

1. **Facial scrub with honey, green tea and sugar**

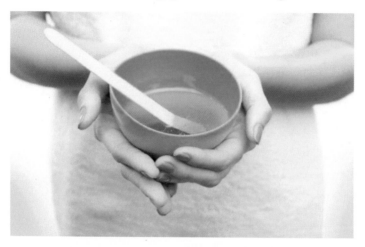

Make green tea and let it become cold. Put one tablespoon of tea in a bowl and add 1 tablespoon of sugar and one tablespoon of honey to it and mix it. That mix will be of thick consistence, but it also depends a lot on the density of the honey. To get a mixture as thick as paste, you add more sugar.

Wash your face and apply this mask. In a circular motion, remove dead cells from the face.

Green tea is great against pimples and acts as a powerful antioxidant. It is good against wrinkles and for skin regeneration. Honey works against bacteria and fungi, so you do natural skin disinfection.

Since honey acts as a kind of preservative, you can store excess of this mixture in the refrigerator for several weeks.

2. *Honey and cinnamon face scrub*

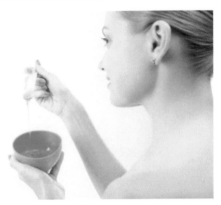

Honey and cinnamon are a powerful combination for weight loss, but also great for removing impurities, bacteria and dead cells of the face. This treatment is great against pimples. <u>You need to mix one teaspoon of cinnamon and one tablespoon of honey in a small bowl to make a paste. Apply to the face by cleaning it in a circular motion.</u> Cinnamon, like honey, fights well with inflammation and pimples and removes dark spots and scars from the face and brightens them.

Since this is also a face mask, do not just rinse the ingredients. Take advantage of them and leave for half an hour and then rinse.

3. *Kefir and oatmeal scrub*

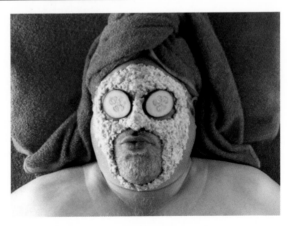

Face scrub is for everyone! :D

Oatmeal delicately softens the face, and kefir is rich in lactic acid and as such an excellent treatment that regenerates skin cells. Mix finely ground oatmeal with a spoonful of kefir. If you do not have kefir, use yogurt. Do the face scrub, but also allow the mask to stay on your skin for 15-20 minutes. It won't hurt. On the contrary, you will like the results!

4. *Sea salt and olive oil face scrub*

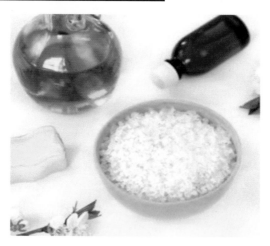

Sea salt is rich in minerals that perfectly regenerate the skin, but make sure it is not bulky. Olive oil is great for skin care, softens it and maintains its elasticity. All you need for this natural face scrub is to mix these two ingredients until you have made a paste. About a tablespoon of salt you should add a tablespoon of olive oil. That's it. Cleanse your face and nourish your skin.

5. *Toothpaste and salt serve your tan!*

Who says with toothpaste you should only brush your teeth? Try it as a face treatment. You need one spoonful of toothpaste, but not the ones that are transparent in the form of gel, but the ones that are not transparent, because it has better abrasive properties. Add one tablespoon of salt to it and make a scrub that will be applied to your face in a circular motion.

6. *Coffee face scrub*

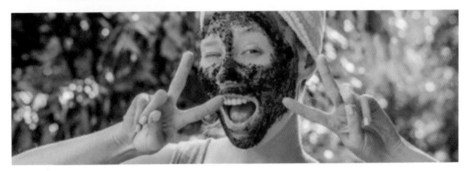

For this treatment all you need is coffee - one tablespoon. To make it in paste form, add one tablespoon of water to it. Apply in a circular motion to your face. Because coffee is good for the skin and promotes surface microcirculation, it is also often used as a treatment for anti-cellulite. After exfoliation, you will notice that your skin is tighter and smoother.

7. *Baking soda face scrub*

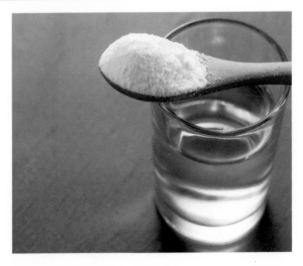

Baking soda is ideal as a scrub because of its slightly grainy structure, but also its ability to soften and nourish the skin. There are several ways to make a baking soda facial scrub. The easiest is the one where you just add water to it and make a paste to rub your face. Plus, you can combine it with coconut or other facial oil. When it comes to coconut oil, add one tablespoon of coconut oil to one tablespoon of baking soda.

8. *Coconut oil and sugar*

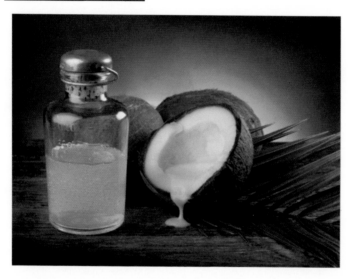

Another of the scrubs combined to combat acne and pimples - coconut oil, sugar and lemon. Coconut oil works against bacteria and fungi, and lemon and sugar soften and nourish the skin and restore its elasticity. Pour a spoonful of sugar into a bowl and add a tablespoon of lemon juice. After that, add the coconut oil until you make a paste.

And this paste in the fridge can take weeks.

9. *Corn Flour Facial Scrub*

Corn flour is one of those ingredients, when in contact with water, will remain in its granular structure, which is what we need when making natural face scrubs. Basic corn flour face treatment involves making a paste with water. <u>However, to enhance the effect of exfoliation, add flour to honey, coconut or olive oil.</u>

10. *Banana for the face*

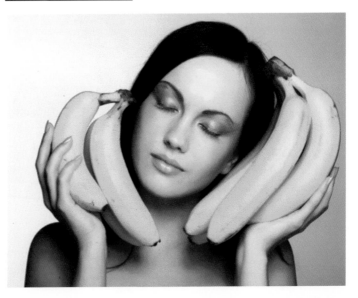

<u>Combine banana and sugar as a face scrub. Simply crush one banana and add a tablespoon of sugar to it.</u> Banana deprives the skin of free radicals and this is a great treatment for wrinkles and premature aging. Not to mention how rich in vitamins and minerals it is. Don't forget to eat one either! And in confidence, banana scrub is my favorite.

11. *Active charcoal for the face*

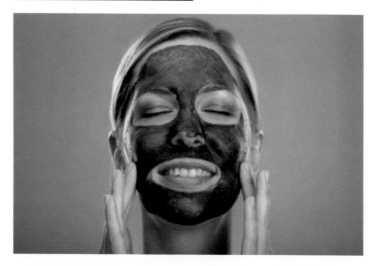

You know those black masks popular in the fight against pimples? They are made on the basis of activated carbon, which is excellent in the fight against toxins. For face use, mix the activated carbon capsule with a spoonful of sugar and a spoonful of olive oil. Cleanse your face with this natural scrub and your skin will shine.

12. *Lavender oil and sugar at bedtime*

If you need a soothing exfoliation after a busy day that relaxes and nourishes the skin and helps you to fall asleep, this is the care you need. Mix a quarter cup of some base oil (olive, coconut), a cup of sugar and 5-6 drops of lavender essential oil. Not only does it smell good, but lavender also has antiseptic properties and this will be a great soothing natural face scrub.

After each facial treatment, whichever of the above recipes you choose, rinse your skin with mild warm water, and finish flushing with cold to close the pores.

Clean your face with a towel, tap movements. Then apply a moisturizer.

There are also scrubs you can buy in stores. More or less, they all do the same thing - they remove a thin layer of skin from the face and the granules they have are crucial in the process. Homemade face scrub that you make yourself is just as effective at it and as you have seen, it can be easily made and you know what you put into it. At least it is natural and homemade!

Scrubs are just part of face care and are not enough on their own, especially for those prone to pimples. What should be applied regularly are natural creams and gels with active ingredients that more effectively address the acne problem.

If you have avoided this treatment so far, I recommend that you try one, right away. If you like sweets, I am sure you have sugar in your house, and you can combine it with some other natural ingredient to make a paste. You will see, your skin is soft and smooth, and you will never neglect this type of care again. Regularly practiced with proper treatment, your pimple problems, if you have them, can become a thing of the past.

Fabulous Skin - How to Keep It?

__Homemade Bath Recipes__

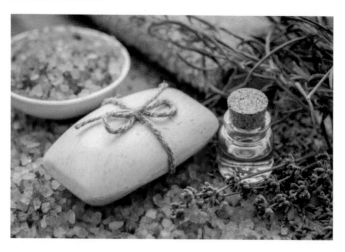

Baths containing natural ingredients can provide our body with many benefits, and a recent study even suggests that immersing your body in warm water could be just as beneficial as exercising, helping to regulate blood sugar!

Not surprisingly, bath is incredibly relaxing. And bath bubbles have therapeutic qualities.

The bath, in general, has existed for centuries. Egyptian, Greek, Chinese and Japanese cultures have benefited from the cosmetic but also therapeutic benefits of the bath.

The comfort that you feel while bathing is thought to be similar to that in the womb, and so it can significantly improve our mood. Research shows that staying in hot water every day for about eight weeks can greatly reduce anxiety - in some cases, perhaps more than taking a prescription drug.

Moreover, baths, especially with homemade baths ingredients, can help with psoriasis, dry skin, better sleep, stimulating brain function, and even helping the body fight off the cold.

Incorporating the right ingredients into your home bath is the key to adding to these benefits!

For example, we know that lavender is probably the most popular essential oil for relaxation.

So read on to find out how you can take a bath with your own homemade recipe. This is a homemade glycerin-free bath, and you can try other essential oils instead of lavender!

How to Make a Homemade Bath?

To make your homemade foam bath, use a container or bottle with an airtight lid and combine almond oil, egg whites and honey. Mix them together well. Light almond oil is perfect to ensure your skin is hydrated, especially if you have dry skin.

Egg White is the key to creating bubbles - although the bubbles may not be as big as the conventional ones you are used to seeing. Honey is a natural humectant, which means it will provide, and help to keep the skin moisturized. It also has antibacterial properties.

Now add Castile soap and essential oils. Castile soap is perfect because it is a completely natural soap that has a vegetable base and is free of chemicals.

Adding a little aromatherapy to your bathing is definitely a plus for the best experience and benefits.

Chamomile essential oil and lavender essential oil are great bathing ingredients as they help fight anxiety and depression.

Mix all ingredients well.

Now that you've made your relaxing bath, it's time to try it out!

Pour 1/4 to 1/2 cup under running water at desired temperature. Keep the remaining amount of bath in the fridge for your next bath!

Ingredients:

- 1/2 cup light almond oil

- 1 egg white

- 1/4 cup of honey

- 1/2 cup Liquid Castile Soap

- 1/2 teaspoon of chamomile essential oil

- 1/2 teaspoon of lavender essential oil

Preparation:

Using a jar or bottle with an airtight lid, mix almond oil, egg whites and honey.

Put them together well.

Add Castile soap and essential oils.

Relax and enjoy all the senses.

It is not difficult to live healthy. You just need to know how!

Natural soaps

Purchasing soaps at their pH value of 9 or 10 can disturb the pH of 5.5 skin, thus allowing bacteria to develop that prevent the natural pH of the skin.

The antibacterial ingredients in soaps are bad for the skin, and more importantly, they are associated with the emergence of antibiotic-resistant bacteria! Fragrances and colors that are added to shopping soaps often cause allergic reactions.

By creating your own natural soap, you can add vegetable oils that will nourish the specific needs of your skin, and with the addition of essential oils and colors, refine the soap and add your own touch of creativity.

For the preparation of natural soap it is necessary to undergo training with an expert. I will provide basic information here, but I emphasize that they are not sufficient for self-production, but you should definitely attend a real soap making workshop.

The raw materials and materials needed to make natural soap are: precise scales, thermometers for liquids, laboratory beakers, plastic spoons, sodium hydroxide (NaOH), vegetable oil, hydrolate or distilled water, or spices with bright colors: pepper, cinnamon, turmeric or for example poppy seeds, and essential oils.

When making soap we need to know the so-called the saponification number - so it should be searched online - for the vegetable oils: ex. for olive oil, it is 0.134, and for palm oil, 0.141.

Principles of Hydrated Hair Care – Simple Homemade Recipes

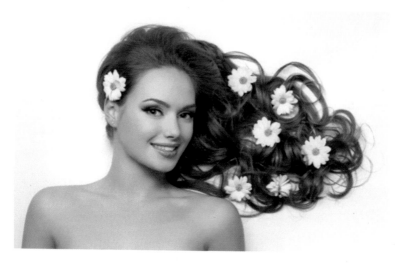

You may be shocked to find that you have simply deprived your hair of moisture all these years in your attempts at having moisturized hair. When you follow these simple rules, hydrated hair isn't far away.

Here is what most people don't know: whether you are using the right oils and other ingredients that soak your hair or scalp healthily, you never need to use a standard shampoo for hair washing - you can use a way gentler, humidifying, or conditioner cleaning process. Use a natural conditioner to remove debris and dust and watch your hair get hydrated rather than you're used. You don't need to necessarily use conditioner on your scalp, so you will not have to scrub your scalp too often if you do use natural oils and other ingredients.

Natural hair care products can sometimes be made at home, and products that can use your hair are probably already in your kitchen.

While probably most of us here have tried the various tricks the internet has to offer and are disappointed with the results, I want to remind you that persistence and regular hair care are essential factors in achieving noticeable results in the long run. Do not give up after the first use of the preparations you have prepared at your home, because you know how people say: ***Rome was not built in a day.***

Below, I offer some completely natural products that have been given by God for the sake of combining healthy and long hair, and I will show you how to nourish your hair with their help.

1. *Coconut oil*

This product really is what you have heard or read at least once - a super-powerful ally, not only for hair care, but also for skin care, makeup removal, and weight loss! If you haven't had one in your house by now, it's a good time to buy one for your bag, and another for the kitchen, because coconut oil is truly a phenomenal food item that will save you money, and make you nicer and more satisfied! Just apply it!

2. *Lemon*

Proven effective tool in combating dull and persistent dandruff! I bet you didn't know that after all those expensive products you were trying to get rid of this little white temptation, the solution lies right in your fridge! The lemon should be squeezed and mixed with a little olive oil, and the mixture should be rubbed into the root of the hair.

Citric acid will eliminate dandruff while oil will treat the scalp. Another tip to combat dandruff: Try to reduce stress and improve nutrition, as these are some of the factors that cause dandruff.

3. *Castor oil*

One of the best natural hair care oils, and one of the strongest factors for hair growth. Castor oil is a bomb in the bottle that will accelerate the growth of your hair from three to five times! In addition, this oil prevents hair loss, and helps fight dandruff. Castor acid helps to balance the pH balance, so castor oil is blogging and also for the health of the scalp.

So, you wonder how to nourish castor oil? Only rub a few drops into the root of the hair. It is advisable to keep your hair moist but not completely wet. You can pour the water into a spray bottle and then spray the root just before applying the oil. Rub slowly, in a circular motion, and repeat the treatment at most twice a week. You can leave it on even overnight (with hair in a towel to avoid greasing the pillow), then rinse with water and shampoo.

Apart from saving you money, these homemade products do not contain any harmful chemicals, so they will not damage your hair and preserve the health of your hair. And this is exactly the path to stunning hair that everyone turns to on the street!

Protect Your Hair!

Now you have put the right ingredients into your hair, and you want to secure your hair with a few more tips of hair care by means of gentle washing, conditioning, and moisturizing. During the day, whether your hair is short or longer, you should avoid to exposure it to bad factors that can damage your hair, like cold, wind, heat and long siting hours on the sun!

It may involve putting the hair in a defensive hairstyle but If you're trying to keep a healthy and stunning look of your hair, the trick is to protect your hair so that over the months and years, it doesn't get shorter and split.

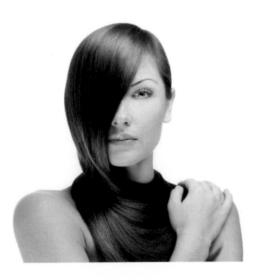

CONCLUSION

Beauty is a woman's privilege. Others are simply born with perfect hair, and some just have to work hard. Yet practically everybody needs to focus on hair to enhance or preserve hair. In this book I provided you with a few tips for handling the crowning glory. I hope you will find a value and benefit from it!

What Did You Think of this Natural Hair Care and Skin Care Guide?

*First of all, I would like to **thank you** for purchasing this book! I am extremely grateful you picked up my book among all the others! I sincerely hope you enjoyed, and I hope you found a value and benefit by reading it.*

I would like to hear from you, and I hope you could take a few minutes of your time to post an honest review on my book page on Amazon. Your feedback and support are very important and it will help me to greatly improve my writing, and make this book even better.

You can post your honest review by click on this link below:

www.amazon.com/review/create-review?&asin=B087NZ81QB
Thank you again for your support!

Printed in Germany
by Amazon Distribution
GmbH, Leipzig

18399562R00063